Assessing the
Contributions of
the Social
Sciences to Health

AAAS Selected Symposia Series

 Published by Westview Press, Inc.
5500 Central Avenue, Boulder, Colorado

for the

 American Association for the Advancement of Science
1776 Massachusetts Avenue, N.W., Washington, D.C.

Assessing the Contributions of the Social Sciences to Health

Edited by
M. Harvey Brenner, Anne Mooney
and Thomas J. Nagy

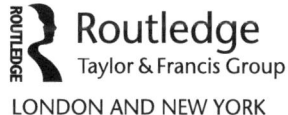

Routledge
Taylor & Francis Group

LONDON AND NEW YORK

First published 1980 by Westview Press

Published 2018 by Routledge
52 Vanderbilt Avenue, New York, NY 10017
2 Park Square, Milton Park, Abingdon, Oxon OX14 4RN

Routledge is an imprint of the Taylor & Francis Group, an informa business

Library of Congress Cataloging in Publication Data
  Main entry under title:
  Assessing the contributions of the social sciences to health.
    (AAAS selected symposium ; 26)
    Bibliography: p.
    1. Social medicine--Congresses. 2. Social medicine--Methodology--
Congresses. 3. Social sciences--Congresses. I. Brenner, Meyer Harvey,
1939-   II. Mooney, Anne. III. Nagy, Thomas J. IV. Series: American
Association for the Advancement of Science. AAAS selected symposium ; 26.
  RA418.A77   362.1   79-24615

ISBN 13: 978-0-367-01770-5 (hbk)
ISBN 13: 978-0-367-16757-8 (pbk)

About the Book

The authors of this book provide a systematic, integrated review and comparison of the contributions of sociology, political science, economics, demography, anthropology, history of science and medicine, psychiatry, and psychology to a number of health-related fields, including epidemiology, health services research, and health policy studies. The book reflects the authors' attitude that multidisciplinary research efforts must be carried out in order to obtain a thorough understanding of the relationship of social science knowledge to health problems.

About the Series

The *AAAS Selected Symposia Series* was begun in 1977 to provide a means for more permanently recording and more widely disseminating some of the valuable material which is discussed at the AAAS Annual National Meetings. The volumes in this *Series* are based on symposia held at the Meetings which address topics of current and continuing significance, both within and among the sciences, and in the areas in which science and technology impact on public policy. The *Series* format is designed to provide for rapid dissemination of information, so the papers are not typeset but are reproduced directly from the camera-copy submitted by the authors, without copy editing. The papers are organized and edited by the symposium arrangers who then become the editors of the various volumes. Most papers published in this *Series* are original contributions which have not been previously published, although in some cases additional papers from other sources have been added by an editor to provide a more comprehensive view of a particular topic. Symposia may be reports of new research or reviews of established work, particularly work of an interdisciplinary nature, since the AAAS Annual Meetings typically embrace the full range of the sciences and their societal implications.

WILLIAM D. CAREY
Executive Officer
American Association for
the Advancement of Science

Contents

Figures and Tables xi

About the Editors and Authors xiii

Overview—*M. Harvey Brenner, Anne Mooney and Thomas J. Nagy* 1

> The Disciplines   5
> *Anthropology, 5; Demography, 5;*
> *Economics, 8; History, 9; Human*
> *Geography, 9; Philosophy, 13;*
> *Political Science, 13; Psychiatry,*
> *15; Psychology, 19; Social Psychol-*
> *ogy, 19; Sociology, 21*
> Cross-Disciplinary Research   21
> The Future   21
> Selected Bibliography   23
> *I. Classics, 23; II. Symposia, 23;*
> *III. Reviews, 24; IV. Epidemiology,*
> *24; V. Health Services Research, 25;*
> *VI. Anthropology, 25; VII. Demography,*
> *26; VIII. Economics, 27; IX. History,*
> *28; X. Human Geography, 30; XI. Philos-*
> *ophy, 31; XII. Political Science, 32;*
> *XIII. Psychiatry, 33; XIV. Psychology,*
> *34; XV. Social Psychology, 35; XVI.*
> *Sociology, 35; XVII. Cross-Disciplin-*
> *ary Research, 36; XVIII. Social Epide-*
> *miological Studies That Include Health*
> *Care, 38*

Part 1 Social, Structural and Demographic Factors

Introduction: Part 1--*John W. Ratcliffe* 41

    The Traditional Health Para-
      digm   41
    The Emergent Paradigm   43
    Notes   47
    References   48

1   Demographic Methods and Their Application
    in the Social and Health Sciences--*Nathan
    Keyfitz* 51

    Acknowledgments   64
    References   64

2   Industrialization and Economic Growth:
    Estimates of Their Effects on the Health
    of Populations--*M. Harvey Brenner* 65

    Overview   65
    Background   67
    Methods   75
    Findings   83
    Conclusions   95
    Appendix I   97
    Appendix II   99
    Appendix III   102
    Appendix IV   107
    Appendix V   109
    Note   111
    References   111

3   Institutional Structure and Process in
    Health Services Innovation: The Reform
    Strategy of the Neighborhood Health
    Center Program--*Jude Thomas May, Katherine
    Knoop Parry, Mary L. Durham and Peter Kong-ming
    New* 117

    Introduction   117
    Purpose of the Paper   119
    The Data   119
    The Strategy and Tactics of
      Institutional Change   120
      Identification of the Problem, 120;
      Formulation of the Problem, 121;
      Operationalizing the Problem, 127

Epilogue: Reform Strategy in
  a Shifting Milieu   132
Conclusion   134
Notes   136
References   138

Part 2   Sociocultural and Psychobiological Dynamics

Introduction: Part 2--*Anne Mooney and Thomas
J. Nagy* 143

4   Cultural and Environmental Factors in
    the Definition and Understanding of
    Health--*Nancie L. Gonzalez* 147

    Notes   157
    References   157

5   The Influence of Psychosocial Factors
    on Susceptibility to Physical Illness--
    William Schofield 159

    References   166

6   Sociocultural and Psychological Aspects
    of the Utilization of Health Services--
    James R. Greenley 169

    Proper Health Care Utilization   170
    Complexities in the Concept of
      Utilization   171
      *Dangers of Aggregating Heteroge-
      neous Utilization Measures, 172*
    Theories of Health Care Utiliz-
      ation   173
      *Decision Points or Stage Models,
      173; "Sets of Variables" Models,
      174; Limitations, Possibilities
      and Alternatives, 174*
    Sociodemographic Correlates of
      Physician Visits   176
    Morbidity and Utilization   177
      *Awareness of Abnormal Bodily
      States, 177; Illness Attributions,
      178; Assessments of Symptoms, 179*
    Income and Utilization   180
      Indices of Access to Care, 182

Subcultural and Ethnic Influ-
    ences   183
Lay Referral and Familial Inter-
action, 184
Knowledge of Illness and Dis-
    ease   185
Beliefs, Attitudes and Utiliz-
    ation   186
Skepticism of Medical Care, 186;
Tendency to Adopt the Sick Role,
188; Other Psychosocial Factors
in Utilization, 190
Psychological Distress and
    Utilization   191
Psychological Distress and the
Etiology of Illness, 192; Psycho-
logical Distress as a Trigger for
Utilization, 192; Psychological
Distress and the Search for Ser-
vices, 193; Physician Response to
Psychological Distress, 194
Conclusion   195
References   197

7   The Bearing of Social Sciences Know-
    ledge on Medical Education and Practice--
    Stanley Joel Reiser 209

    Notes   215
    References   215

Figures and Tables

Overview

Table 1   Anthropology   4

Table 2   Demography   6

Table 3   Economics   7

Table 4   History   10

Table 5   Human Geography   11

Table 6   Philosophy   12

Table 7   Political Science   14

Table 8   Psychiatry   16

Table 9   Psychology   17

Table 10   Social Psychology   18

Table 11   Sociology   20

Chapter 1

Table 1   Percent increase in expectation
               of life   56

Chapter 2

Table 1   Multiple regression equations of
               national economic indices on age-
               specific mortality rates   80

Table 2   Relationships between unemploy-
                 ment and mortality rates   84

Table 3   Multiple regression equations of
                 national economic indices on
                 age-specific mortality rates   86

Figure 1   Relation between mortality and
                 employment rates, ages 55-64;
                 detrended residual plot   .   90

Figure 2   Relation between mortality and
                 employment rates, ages 55-64;
                 three-year moving averages of
                 annual changes   92

Figure 3   Relation between mortality and
                 employment rates, ages 65-74   93

Figure 4   Relation between mortality and
                 employment rates, ages 75-84   94

Chapter 3

Table 1   Types of neighborhood health center-
                 sponsoring institutions   133

About the Editors and Authors

M. Harvey Brenner, *associate professor in the Division of Operations Research and the Department of Behavioral Sciences at Johns Hopkins University, specializes in the sociology of medicine and psychiatry.* He has published *articles on trends in alcohol consumption and cirrhosis mortality, and on correlations between economic changes and heart disease mortality and fetal, infant, and maternal mortality.* He is the author of Mental Illness and the Economy *(Harvard University Press, 1973) and* Estimating the Social Costs of National Economic Policy: Implications for Mental and Physical Health and Criminal Aggression *(Report for the Joint Economic Committee of Congress; U.S. Government Printing Office, 1976).*

Anne Mooney, *assistant professor at the University of Delaware College of Urban Affairs and Public Policy and Department of Sociology, is currently a postdoctoral fellow in the Division of Operations Research at Johns Hopkins School of Hygiene and Public Health.* Her work focuses on *social epidemiology, urbanization and health, and health indices, and she is a member of the Jefferson Center for the Study of Alcoholism, Jefferson Medical College.* She has *published articles on measuring health levels for community health planning and on epidemiology of alcoholism and alcohol abuse, and is coeditor of* Health Goals and Health Indicators: Policy, Planning and Evaluation *(with J. Elinson and A. Seigmann; Westview/AAAS, 1977).*

Thomas J. Nagy, *a postdoctoral fellow in the Operations Research Division of Johns Hopkins University School of Hygiene and Public Health, is studying the effects of the economy on social and medical pathology and on measurement of intervention effects.* He was a research fellow at the Center for the Study of Law and Society at the University of

California-Berkeley and has published articles on evaluation, replication and the economy and on psychopharmacology and criminality. He is coauthor of Predictive Sentencing: An Empirical Evaluation *(with L. H. Whinery et al.; Lexington, 1976).*

Mary L. Durham, *assistant research sociologist in the Department of Psychiatry at the University of California at Los Angeles, is a specialist in the field of medical sociology. She is the author of several articles on neighborhood health centers.*

Nancie L. Gonzalez *is vice chancellor for academic affairs and professor of anthropology at the University of Maryland, College Park. A cultural anthropologist by training, she has done field work in Guatemala, Dominican Republic, and the Southwestern United States, is past president of the Society for Applied Anthropology, and is a council member of the American Association for the Advancement of Science. She is the editor of* Social and Technological Management in Dry Lands: Past and Present, Indigenous and Imposed *(AAAS Selected Symposium No. 10, Westview, 1978) and the author of numerous articles on the anthropology of health and disease.*

James R. Greenley, *associate professor in the Department of Psychiatry and Sociology at the University of Wisconsin-Madison, is a medical sociologist. He has published articles on social selection processes leading to psychiatric care, user satisfaction with health services, and organizational factors affecting access to services.*

Nathan Keyfitz *is Andelot Professor of Sociology and Demography and chairman of the Department of Sociology at Harvard University. A member of the National Academy of Sciences and of the American Academy of Arts and Sciences, he is also a fellow of the Royal Statistical Society, the Royal Society of Canada, and the American Statistical Association, and a former president of the Population Association of America. He is editor of* Theoretical Population Biology, *and his many publications include* Applied Mathematical Demography *(Wiley, 1977) and* Causes of Death: Life Tables for National Populations *(with S. H. Preston and R. Schoen; Seminar Press, 1972).*

Jude Thomas May, *associate professor in the Department of Social Sciences and Health Behavior at the University of Oklahoma Health Sciences Center, specializes in the sociology of health and medicine. She is coauthor of several articles and a book,* Neighborhood Health Center Program *(National Association of Community Health Centers, Inc., and the National Urban Coalition, 1976), and* The Neighborhood Health Center Movement: A Social Analysis of Policy Formulation and Innovation in Health Services *(in process).*

Peter Kong-ming New, *a professor in the Department of Behavioral Science at the University of Toronto, specializes in medical sociology and anthropology. He is a former chairman of the Medical Sociology Section of the American Sociological Association, a member of the Executive Committee of the Society for Applied Anthropology, and of the National Health Advisory Committee of Health and Welfare Canada, and serves on the Professional Advisory Board of the Addiction Research Foundation, Ontario. He has published numerous papers on topics such as citizen participation in neighborhood health centers and mental health administration, and he is an associate editor of* Human Organization, Sociological Quarterly *and* Sociology of Health and Illness.

Katherine Knoop Parry, *doctoral candidate in the Department of Social Science and Health Behavior at the University of Oklahoma Health Sciences Center, is specializing in medical anthropology and sociology.*

John W. Ratcliffe *is currently director of the Program in Population and Health Policy and associate professor in the Graduate School of Public and International Affairs at the University of Pittsburgh. A specialist in health education, he is the author of* Population Control vs. Social Justice: Population Policies and the Political Economy *(New York Monthly Review Press, 1979) and of articles on the relationship between social justice and health, population change, and population and development in Kerala, India. He has served as population and health specialist with the World Bank's New Delhi office (1972-75) and as chief advisor to the Ford Foundation's population research and training project in East Pakistan (now Bangladesh).*

Stanley Joel Reiser, *a physician, is assistant professor and director of the Program in the History of Medicine, Harvard Medical School. He is a member of the Board of Advisors in the Harvard Medical School, and was director of the Interdisciplinary Study Group of Health Care Policy at the Kennedy Institute of Politics. He is the author of* Medicine and the Reign of Technology *(Cambridge University Press, 1978) and coeditor of* Ethics in Medicine: Historical Perspectives and Contemporary Concerns *(with A. Dyck and W. Curran; MIT Press, 1977).*

William Schofield, *professor in the Department of Psychiatry and Psychology at the University of Minnesota, is a clinical psychologist. He is past chairman of the American Psychological Association's Task Force on Health Research (1973-75) and a fellow of the APA, and chairman of the Minnesota Psychological Association's Committee on Ethics. His publications include* Psychotherapy: The Purchase of Friendship *(Prentice-Hall, 1964).*

M. Harvey Brenner, Anne Mooney,
Thomas J. Nagy

Overview

The purpose of this volume is to examine from a multidisciplinary perspective the contributions of the social sciences to knowledge about health. We mean by health what is usually called health status or, for population aggregates, health levels--that is, measures of mortality, morbidity, disability, and impairment of function. This overview defines the field of interest, both conceptually and operationally, through a taxonomy of disciplines and subdisciplines and a selective list of references to writings in the field. The papers, in turn, review more intensively some of the main literatures of social science that relate to health--giving an expert author's particular emphasis, assessment, and outlook.

The actual and potential contributions of social science to health have long been recognized. Half a century ago in the United States, for example, three classic works were published within a five-year period: Dublin's Health and Wealth, Sydenstricker's Health and Environment, and the often-cited final report of the Committee on the Costs of Medical Care, Medical Care for the American People (Selected Bibliography, page 23, Part I). More recently, a considerable literature of research reports, monographs, reviews, and symposia dealing with health issues from the perspectives of the social sciences has developed. Among the symposia we find a few attempts at broad coverage, but most tend to be oriented around one specific topic or problem or to involve only one or two disciplines. Typical of recent symposia of relatively broad scope are those listed in Part II (page 23) of the bibliography.

This volume is distinctive for its focus on health, its inclusion of a broad range of disciplines, and its focus on review and assessment. Considered review of the contributions of social sciences in health research is a timely, if difficult, undertaking since the previous comprehensive reviews were published 15 to 20 years ago (Selected Bibliography, page 24, Part III). Furthermore, the emphasis on presentation of the state of the art in each of several disciplines means that specialists in those areas will likely find little that is fundamentally new with respect to their own fields. Rather we expect that social, medical, and biological scientists will find a useful introduction to the scope and contributions of each of the various social sciences--apart from their own fields of expertise--as these relate to health.

Social research has identified three broad effects of sociocultural conditions on health. In the first instance, the matter of how health is defined in any society is itself an aspect of culture, as are the behaviors usually associated with roles wholly or partially determined by an individual's health status. Historically, as social epidemiologists consistently report, socioeconomic variables appear to have had the predominant impact on changing health levels in populations. A third domain of social science concern with health is in matters of policy--efforts intended to influence health levels by means of alterations in the availability of medical care and in social, economic and political conditions. These areas may also be described by framing the types of questions about health for which social scientists have offered theoretical, methodological, or empirical contributions.

I.   In a particular society or culture, what is meant by health and illness, what is believed about these states or conditions, and what behavioral practices surround them?

II. What causal factors account for the levels of health and the patterns of illness in a population?

III. What are the organizational or policy measures by which the society attempts to alter the levels of health and distribution of illness?

It is important to point out that we exclude the very significant social science contributions to the literatures on the internal organization and administration of health-care services, the history of the medical profession, the sociology of health-care occupations, or the economics of the health-care industry. While these studies represent some of the most sophisticated research in the existing social science literature, they do not generally deal with the impact of organizational matters on health levels.

On the other hand, the influence of the social sciences in health has not been confined to work of persons trained in and identified with the social sciences themselves. The public health fields of epidemiology and health services research, corresponding respectively to our questions II and III, both use methods and theories developed in the social sciences. Reference to representative items from these two literatures should therefore be included in any review of social science contributions to health (Selected Bibliography, pages 24-25, Parts IV and V).

It may be asked since these are fields within public health and not traditional social science disciplines or subdisciplines, what makes them social science? It is because their theories are derived from social science, some or all of their independent variables are likewise, and their methods are social science research methods. Examples of the theories are complex organizations, networks, and social support. Examples of variables are social class, personality type, and gross national product. Examples of the third are survey techniques, scaling of variables, and multivariate methods of data analysis.

The seven papers in this volume were presented at the 1978 AAAS Symposium on "Assessing the Contributions of the Social Sciences to Health." The papers were not meant to be comprehensive reviews of the major research efforts of all of the social sciences insofar as they bear on health. Rather, the authors were asked to select what they thought to be the most prominent issues in their respective fields of study as they relate to health. They were then to review the fields critically with the objective of coming to some conclusion as to their overall contribution. In some cases, the authors attempted to summarize their field's progress, while in others the authors went beyond summary to present original formulations, or formal theoretical models, based upon those summaries. Each paper also provides an orientation toward the future--in terms of either appropriate or probable directions of research or applications to policy.

While the symposium papers do deal in depth with many of the most significant areas of social science research on health, the editors decided it would be worthwhile to present the reader with an overall outline of social science contributions to knowledge about health and illness. In this introduction we have therefore briefly outlined the types of health-related research that have been traditional in each of eleven disciplines: anthropology, demography, economics, history, human geography, philosophy, political science, psychiatry, psychology, social psychology, and sociology.

For each discipline, we have devised a table which indicates as many as possible of the topics, both analytical and substantive, on which specialized literatures exist that have

Table 1. Anthropology

Conceptualization	Epidemiology	Societal Response
Analytic Subfields		
Social Anthropology Cultural Anthropology Linguistics	Social Anthropology Cultural Anthropology Physical Anthropology Archeology	Social Anthropology Cultural Anthropology Linguistics Archeology
Topical Categories		
Definitions of Health, Illness, Disease Beliefs and Practices Magic, Science and Religion	Effects of Environment on Health Social Organization of Health and Illness Sociobiology Economic Anthropology Diet and Nutrition	Beliefs and Practices Social Organization of Health and Illness Role of Healer Magic, Science and Religion Diet and Nutrition

direct relevance to health issues. The upper panel gives
elements of an intrinsic structure found in the theoretical
foundations of the field, while the lower panel shows the
empirical structure of the field--the actual themes and subjects of research. The topics are listed according to the
large questions--cultural, epidemiological, or policy--to
which they are pertinent.

The Disciplines

Anthropology

The field of anthropology is among the substantively
more comprehensive of the social sciences. This breadth
is reflected in the range of literature covering all the basic
questions addressed by the social sciences in health and covering many of the societies of the world, past and present
(Table 1; Selected Bibliography, page 25).

The fields of social and cultural anthropology are concerned with the relationship of humans to their environment
as organized and mediated by social structure and culture. As
indicated in Table 1, these subfields may be concerned with
any of the three key issues. Physical anthropology, concerned
as it is with the effects of culture and society on anatomi-
cal and other physical characteristics of populations, contributes to appreciation of the effects of diet, nutrition,
climate, and other aspects of environment as they impinge on
health status. Linguistics focuses attention on the vocabu-
lary and meanings attached to particular states of health and,
indeed, on the very concepts of health, illness, and disease
themselves. Archeological studies provide a particular
framework and set of methodologies to learn for nonliving
societies what cultural and physical anthropologists study
in living societies.

An indication of the range of substantive topics dealt
with in these fields is shown in the lower panel of the table.
Further elaboration may be found in the paper by Gonzalez in
this volume.

Demography

Demography is often thought to be a subfield of sociology,
although much demographic research is in fact done by persons
trained in economics, anthropology, statistics, medicine,
and other fields. The field is fundamental to social scientific studies in both epidemiology and health policy, since
it deals with size, distribution, structure, and change in
populations--characteristics analytically understood to be

Table 2. Demography

Conceptualization	Epidemiology	Societal Response
	Analytic Subfields	
---	Population Size and Distribution	Population Size and Distribution
	Population Structure	Population Structure
	Population Change	Population Change
	Topical Categories	
---	Paleodemography	Population Policy
	Historical Demography	Social Demography
	Social Demography	Historical Demography
	Health Status	Health Status
	Measurement	Measurement

Table 3. Economics

Conceptualization	Epidemiology	Societal Response
	Analytic Subfields	
---	Economic Growth Econometrics	Public Finance Welfare Economics Income and Employment Theory Economic Policy International Trade Relations Labor Economics Operations Research and Systems Analysis Econometrics Economic Growth
	Topical Categories	

---	Effects of Health on
	    Economic Growth
	Industrial Pollution
	Nutrition
	Effects of Economy on
	    Health
		Financing of Health Care
		Costs of Health Care
		Production of Health
		    Care Services
		Allocation of Health
		    Care Resources
		Demand for Health and
		    Health Care

determined by natality, mortality, nuptiality, and mobility
(Table 2; Selected Bibliography, page 26).

The traditional approach of demography to measurement
and analysis of health status is through mortality studies,
using the life table as an analytic tool and expressing health
in terms of death rates and expectation of life at various
ages, as Keyfitz describes in Chapter 1 of this volume. The
bibliographic materials show, however, that recently attention
has also been focused on the interrelationships between
health levels and the rates of fertility, marriage, and migration, as well as population size, density, structure, and
change. Keyfitz's paper also shows that demographic work
can aid in appreciation of the effects of population characteristics and demographic processes on the evaluation of
alternative health research policies.

Considerable interest in the sociological question of
the relationship of health to social status is supported by
demographic materials and analyses that allow systematic
measurement of that relationship. Likewise, economic questions related to health can be examined using basic demographic
data in combination with economic measures. (See, for example,
Brenner's paper in this volume.) For whole populations, therefore, demographic data, measurements, and analyses are all
of importance to other social science fields and to interdisciplinary work.

Economics

Economists study the allocation of limited resources
among unlimited and competing demands. The field is divided
theoretically into macro-economics, which examines the problem
of full use of resources at the national level, and micro-eco-
nomics, which deals with the allocation of resources by single
units--either individuals or organizations studied as though
they were individuals (Table 3; Selected Bibliography, page 27).

Health economics has typically focused on quantifying
over time the resources used in health services delivery, the
organization and financing of health services, and the efficiency of the allocation and use of resources for health purposes, including the effects of preventive, curative, and re-
habilitative services on individual and national productivity.
Most work relating the economy and health has used health
levels to account for economic development. Few researchers
have sought to account for changes in health by examining
changes in the economy.

Generally, health economics has been relatively insulated from other social science disciplines. Economics is, however, linked with history of illness and with demography through the field of economic history. In addition, when economists use political, legal, and other social factors as explanatory variables, rather than treating them as constants, they intersect with political science and sociology.

History

History, along with prehistoric archeology and historical demography, documents the past and analyzes relationships between the social environment of historical populations and their health status levels. These studies may focus on either epidemiologic or policy questions. In addition, historians determine the matters of fact and chronology that constitute data on the basis of which other social scientists carry out further analyses (Table 4; Selected Bibliography, page 28).

As we have already suggested, historical epidemiology serves to illuminate the effects of technological change and economic development on health levels. Historical methods and materials at present constitute a largely untapped resource for epidemiologic research on chronic diseases and for evaluation of health policies in populations where mortality from infectious disease is largely controlled. Studies of the invention and diffusion of medical science, institutions, preventive practices, and treatments make possible an evaluation of public health and medical care policies. Reiser's paper in this volume treats the diffusion of social science into medicine and medical education.

Human Geography

Human geography brings into the social science arsenal the most thorough measurement and analysis of spatial characteristics of human environments, organizations, and behaviors. This concern and skill are manifest in such activities as mapping of disease, epidemiologic studies of the spatial and temporal relationship between disease and characteristics of the population or the environment, and studies of the location of health care services in relationship to population. Geographers treat epidemiologic problems in spatial terms and in relationship to the natural and human environments; they treat location, availability, and access to health services in the same terms (Table 5; Selected Bibliography, page 30).

Geographic work overlaps extensively with sociology, demography, and anthropology, and all of the geographic

Table 4. History

Conceptualization	Epidemiology	Societal Response
	Analytic Subfields	
---	History of Medicine Social History Economic History	History of Medicine Social History Intellectual History Economic History
	Topical Categories	
---	History of Illness History of Public Health and Personal Health Practices	Historiography History of Illness History of Public Health and Personal Health Practices History of Medical Science and Technology History of Policy History of Health History of Institutions and Professions

Table 5. Human Geography

Conceptualization	Epidemiology	Societal Response
	Analytic Subfields	
---	Social Geography	Social Geography
	Cultural Geography	Cultural Geography
	Economic Geography	Economic Geography
	Political Geography	Political Geography
	Topical Categories	
---	Spatial Epidemiology	Patient Travel
	Disease Ecology	Location of Services
	Disease Diffusion	Nutrition Policy
	Disease Mapping	Behavioral Aspects of
	Diet and Nutrition	Health and Illness
	Cultural and Ecological	
	Studies	
	Behavioral Aspects of	
	Health and Illness	

Table 6. Philosophy

Conceptualization	Epidemiology	Societal Response
Analytic Subfields		
Ethics	Philosophy of Science	Ethics
Philosophy of Religion		Philosophy of Religion
Philosophy of Law		Philosophy of Science
Philosophy of Science		Philosophy of Social Science
Philosophy of Social Science		Philosophy of Law
		Social Philosophy
Topical Categories		
Behavior Control	Social Science Methodology	Behavior Control
Values, Ethics, and Technology	• Indicators	Codes of Professional Ethics
Death and Dying	• Concepts	Medical Ethics Education
Genetics, Fertilization, and Birth	• Causal relations	Values, Ethics, and Technology
		Death and Dying
		Experimentation and Consent
		Genetics, Fertilization, and Birth
		Health Care Delivery
		Population and Birth Control
		Scarce Medical Resources
		Truth-Telling in Medicine
		Confidentiality
		Health Policy Planning

measurements and methods have some applications as well in economic and historical studies. It is clear from the existence of such subfields of study as economic geography and social geography that considerable influence has already occurred between pairs of disciplines. Pyle's (1977) article suggests some of the additional contributions that geography may make to health studies.

Philosophy

Philosophy is not, of course, usually considered a social scientific discipline. There are a variety of good reasons, however, for bringing it explicitly into the purview of this volume. Most generally, logical, epistemological, and metaphysical questions may all usefully be posed with respect to the work of social scientists in the health field. These questions can help to illuminate similarities and differences among the fields that may not be obvious to scientists working in the fields; they can then show under what circumstances differences are resolvable or not (Table 6; Selected Bibliography, page 31).

More concretely, social and political philosophy underlie much of sociological and political science. Some of the implications for social scientific analyses and policy recommendations are elaborated by Ratcliffe in his introduction to the first part of this volume. In addition, particular modes of doing scientific analysis--as explicated by the philosophy of science--underlie statistical theories and techniques. For discussion of some of these issues, readers are referred to the Science symposium.

Finally, still more concretely, many of the current issues in social science and biomedicine are ethical issues with which philosophers are better equipped to deal by training in critical thinking, if not by substantive familiarity with the problem. Again, natural alliances between and among fields are supported by the practical problems that no one field is fully equipped to handle.

The bibliography of bioethics published by the Hastings Center provides the categories that were adapted for Table 6.

Political Science

The contributions of political science to the enterprise fall most heavily in the definitions and policy areas, (1) the official, legitimate, public definitions of health and illness that are supported by agencies of government, and (2) the policies by which modern societies carry out their public

Table 7. Political Science

Conceptualization	Epidemiology	Societal Response
Analytic Subfields		
Public Law Public Administration Policy Analysis	Political Theory Public Law Regulation	Political Theory Political Behavior Policy Analysis Public Law Public Administration
Topical Categories		

Civil Rights and
  Civil Liberties
Health Policy Analysis
	Occupational Safety and
	  Health Policy
	Environmental Policy
		Comparative and Inter-
		  national Health Policy
		Consumer-Provider
		  Relations
		Costs and Financing
		Health Care Organization
		Health Planning
		Malpractice and Liability
		Professions and Manpower
		Health Policy Analysis

health-related activities. The first of these is important
in determination of such questions as who is legally ill,
physically or mentally, and what are the consequences for this
person's other civil and social rights and responsibilities.
The second has to do with organization and investment of resources to improve health levels, decrease suffering, and improve expectation of life--either by preventive or therapeutic
measures (Table 7; Selected Bibliography, page 32).

Political analyses may be carried out at many levels of
geographical or administrative units from comparative/inter-
national to city or neighborhood levels. (See, for example,
the paper by May et al. in this volume.) In institutional
terms, they may deal with the development and determination of
policy, the administrative implementation of policy, and the
settlement of disputes in the judicial system. It would appear that in the past the first two have been particularly
emphasized, but many unresolved ethical issues have made the
judicial system increasingly prominent.

The categories in Table 7 were adapted from the bibliog-
raphies published by the Journal of Health Politics, Policy
and Law.

Psychiatry

Psychiatry, now perhaps attempting to become the quintes-
sential behavioral science, was once understood more narrowly
as the medical specialty which prevents or treats mental disorder. The field presently deals with the stressful consequences of disturbances in the social environment as these
are manifest in all kinds of pathological conditions, not only
mental illness and behavioral problems (Table 8; Selected
Bibliography, page 33).

All three issues areas come into the purview of psychiatric research and practice. In development of diagnostic
criteria and classificatory schemes, psychiatry shares the
definitional task with psychology and to some extent anthropology and philosophy. Psychiatric epidemiology uses the
standard tools of epidemiology, but is notable for having
developed community survey instruments for estimation of
prevalence of mental disorder and psychiatric registers for
assessing both general utilization patterns and the course of
treated mental disorder over long periods. Policy alternatives
may be derived from epidemiologic studies, but treatment evaluation, broadly construed, constitutes perhaps an even more
important contribution of psychiatry to policy.

Table 8. Psychiatry

Conceptualization	Epidemiology	Societal Response
	Analytic Subfields	
Neurology	Psychiatric Epidemiology	Neurology
Nosology		Pharmacology
Psychodiagnosis		Psychotherapy
	Topical Categories	
Child Psychiatry	Case-Finding	Planning
Adolescent Psychiatry	Epidemiologic Surveys	Administration
Geriatric Psychiatry	Psychiatric Registers	Evaluation of Treatment
Forensic Psychiatry	Community Psychiatry	Psychoanalysis
	Social Factors in Disorder	Psychotherapy
	Social Context of Disorder	Chemotherapy
	Developmental Psychiatry	Psychosurgery

Table 9. Psychology

Conceptualization	Epidemiology	Societal Response
	Analytic Subfields	
	Developmental Psychology	Clinical Psychology
	Personality	Counselling Psychology
	Motivational Psychology	Learning Theory
	Topical Categories	
	Stress	Behavior Modification
	Life-Cycle Stages	Counseling
	Personality Types	Psychotherapy
	Individual Differences	Group Therapy
		Therapeutic Community
		Individualization of Treatment
		Evaluation of Treatment
Scaling		
Typologies		
Test Construction		
Diagnosis		
Health Status Measurement		
Objective Testing		
Projective Testing		

Table 10. Social Psychology

Analytic Subfields

Conceptualization	Epidemiology	Societal Response
Attitudes, Values, and Beliefs	Socialization	Socialization
Influence and Persuasion	Mass Communications	Mass Communications
Attribution	Labeling Theory	Attitudes, Values and Beliefs
Labeling Theory		Influence and Persuasion
		Small Groups
		Political Behavior
		Consumer Behavior
		Social Movements
		Labeling Theory

Topical Categories

Conceptualization	Epidemiology	Societal Response
Labeling of Deviance	Advertising	Evaluation of Health Education
Health Beliefs and Values	Diffusion of Innovations	Diffusion of Innovations
	Social Support and Stress	Organization of Health Services
		Self-help groups
		Group Therapy
		Socialization into Health Professions
		Utilization of Health Services

Psychology

Psychology, like psychiatry, and unlike the other social sciences, has a pronounced clinical orientation. Social psychology, which appears as a separate discipline in this scheme, is viewed by some as a subfield of psychology; both share an interest in the way that human attachments and exposure to communications change health attitudes and behaviors. A concern for definitions of illness and classifications of symptoms is shared by psychology with psychiatry (Table 9; Selected Bibliography, page 34).

Among the fields of psychology, psychological testing and diagnosis conceptualize and operationalize definitions of mental conditions, including illness; individual psychology probes the distribution of mental illness based on experiential, personality and motivational factors; and behavior modification seeks to alter deranged behavior, to increase patient compliance with prescribed medical regimens, and to teach and maintain health-promoting behaviors.

Some of the most interesting and important recent epidemiological research contributed by the fields of psychology and psychiatry is reviewed and discussed in detail by Schofield in a paper in this volume. The key issues around which this work focuses are the role of stress and of personality type in the etiology and course of illnesses.

Social Psychology

Social psychology probes the ways in which individuals interact, communicate, and influence each other by examining how individuals affect the social process and how intrapsychic states and personality are influenced by social processes. Understanding these processes of simultaneous interaction is critical both to strategies for compliance to medical regimens and also to the dissemination of public health programs. Further, much disease is understood to be the product of interpersonal and social forces or is affected by these forces (Table 10; Selected Bibliography, page 35).

The definitional problem is addressed in social psychology by studies of labeling and attribution. (See the paper by Greenley in this volume.) The distribution of illness is viewed as the product of both socialization to health attitudes, values, and beliefs and the tendency to adopt the sick role, as well as the product of advertising which influences the rate of diffusion of healthy and unhealthy practices. Other concerns of social psychology in health are the development of professional roles and the content, process and productivity of both work groups and therapy groups.

Table 11. Sociology

Conceptualization	Epidemiology	Societal Response
	Analytic Subfields	
Social Organization	Social Organization	Social Organization
	Sociology of Groups	Sociology of Groups
	Human Ecology	Human Ecology
	Topical Categories	
Culture	Stratification	Formal Organizations and
Sociology of Religion	Social Epidemiology	Bureaucracy
Health Beliefs and	Urban Sociology	Occupations and Professions
Practices	Race and Ethnic	Political Sociology
	Relations	Urban Sociology
	Culture and Personality	Sociology of the Family
		Race and Ethnic Relations
		Economy and Society
		Culture and Personality

Sociology

Medical sociology is a well-developed subfield of sociology; many of its concerns were also discussed in the social psychology section. The sociology considered here is the core of the discipline--the study of social organization--in relationship to health. This organization influences both the epidemiology of illness and health and the characteristics of the formal and informal social mechanisms for dealing with health-related conditions (Table 11; Selected Bibliography, page 35).

Probably the most important question that sociologists, as well as some other social scientists, have dealt with over the years is the differential in health levels by social characteristics. With the advent of more nearly universal access to health care in the most developed of modern societies, as described in Greenley's paper, many observers thought that such differentials--at least by social status--should disappear. Since that has not turned out to be the case, efforts are now underway to reconceptualize the relationship in epidemiologic terms, drawing on research in several of the social sciences, including social psychology and psychiatry.

Cross-Disciplinary Research

We have noted in several instances that the distinctions among social science disciplines are not clear cut; many problems, theories, concepts, and methods overlap pairs or triads of these fields. Furthermore, it is increasingly recognized that no one discipline is equipped to deal adequately with many of the policy issues to which social science speaks. These circumstances have given rise over the years to much cross-disciplinary research and colloquy, as social scientists attempt to expand their perspectives and sharpen their insights. Examples of some recent efforts in cross-disciplinary review and synthesis are found in the bibliography (page 36). These works provide some of the richest insights and innovative analyses of social science research in health.

The Future

The reader may have observed that one major area of health research is conspicuous by its virtual absence from the social science literature. This area concerns the examination of effects of treatment. It is indeed curious that while the social epidemiology of illness and of health care utilization are quite large, with rare exceptions (see Bibliography, page 38) there is practically no social science

tradition of systematic analysis of the impact of treatment
of characteristics of patients. The relative absence of such
a research literature is especially difficult to justify,
since precisely the same summary and analytic tools that are
used in epidemiology can be used in evaluation of patient
care. Perhaps part of the reason for the paucity of such
research is to be found in Keyfitz's paper, which suggests
that epidemiology is frequently thought to be pertinent only
to the discovery of the etiology of disease, rather than to
the course of particular diseases.

It is precisely in the area of treatment evaluation that
social epidemiology can make contributions that are closest
to the immediate interests of clinicians. There is little
doubt in our minds that the introduction of this type of
social science contribution to health is only a matter of
time. Moreover,it is possible that through contributions in
this area social science research may eventually find itself
in the mainstream of the medical school curriculum.

Selected Bibliography

Part I. Classics

Committee on the Costs of Medical Care. Medical Care for the American People. The Final Report of the Committee on the Costs of Medical Care. Chicago: University of Chicago Press, 1932.

Dublin, Louis I. Health and Wealth: A Survey of the Economics of World Health. New York: Harper & Brothers, 1928.

Sydenstricker, Edgar. Health and Environment. New York: McGraw-Hill Book Company, Inc., 1933.

Part II. Symposia

Elinson, Jack, Anne Mooney, and Athilia E. Siegman, eds. Health Goals and Health Indicators: Policy, Planning and Evaluation. AAAS Selected Symposium 2. Boulder, Colorado: Westview Press, for the American Association for the Advancement of Science, 1977.

Health Maintenance. Science 200: 4344(26 May 1978): 845-981.

Jaco, E. Gartly, ed. Patients, Physicians and Illness: A Sourcebook of Behavioral Science and Health. 2d ed. New York: The Free Press, 1972.

Katz, Alfred H. and Jean Spencer Felton, eds. Health and the Community: Readings in the Philosophy and Sciences of Public Health. New York: The Free Press, 1965.

Knowles, John H., ed. Doing Better and Feeling Worse: Health in the United States. New York: W.W. Norton & Company, Inc., 1977.

Lewis, Charles E., Rashi Fein, and David Mechanic. A Right to Health: The Problem of Access to Primary Medical Care. New York: John Wiley & Sons, 1976.

Part III. Reviews

Anderson, Odin W. and Milvoy S. Seacat. "Behavioral
Science Research in the Health Field: A Statement of
Problems and Priorities." Social Problems 6:3 (Winter
1958-59): 268-271.

Polgar, Steven. "Health and Human Behavior: Areas of
Interest Common to the Social and Medical Sciences."
Current Anthropology 3:2 (April 1962): 159-205.

Saunders, Lyle. "The Contributions and Limitations of
Behavioral Science in Public Health." Health and the
Community: Readings in the Philosophy and Sciences of
Public Health, Alfred H. Katz and Jean Spencer Felton,
eds. New York: The Free Press, 1965, pp. 567-582.

Part IV. Epidemiology

Cassel, John. "Social Science Theory as a Source of
Hypotheses in Epidemiological Research." American
Journal of Public Health 54 (September 1964): 1482-1488.

Fox, John P., Carrie E. Hall, and Lila Elveback.
Epidemiology: Man and Disease. New York: Macmillan,
1970.

Lilienfeld, Abraham M. Foundations of Epidemiology.
New York: Oxford University Press, 1976.

MacMahon, Brian and Thomas F. Pugh. Epidemiology:
Principles and Methods. Boston: Little Brown, 1970.

Mausner, Judith S. and Anita K. Bahn. Epidemiology:
An Introductory Text. Philadelphia: W.B. Saunders Company,
1974.

Susser, Mervyn. Causal Thinking in the Health Sciences:
Concepts and Strategies of Epidemiology. New York:
Oxford University Press, 1973.

Part V. Health Services Research

Arnold, Mary F., L. Vaughn Blankenship, and John M. Hess, eds. Administering Health Systems: Issues and Perspectives. Chicago: Aldine Publishing Company, 1971.

Bailey, Norman T.J. and Mark Thompson. System Aspects of Health Planning. New York: American Elsevier Publishing Co., 1975.

Blum, Henrik L. Expanding Health Care Horizons: From a General Systems Concept of Health to a National Health Policy. Oakland, California: Third Party Associates, 1976.

Donabedian, Avedis. Aspects of Medical Care Administration: Specifying Requirements for Health Care. Cambridge: Published for the Commonwealth Fund by Harvard University Press, 1973.

Hyman, Herbert H. Health Planning -- A Systematic Approach. Germantown, Maryland: Aspen Systems Corporation, 1976.

McLaughlin, Curtis P. and Alan Sheldon. The Future and Medical Care. Cambridge: Ballinger Publishing Company, 1974.

White, Paul E. and George J. Vlasak, eds. Interorganizational Research in Health: Conference Proceedings. Washington: National Center for Health Services Research, 1970.

Part VI. Anthropology

Ackerknecht, Erwin H. Medicine and Ethnology: Selected Essays. H.H. Walser and H.M. Koelbing, eds. Baltimore: The Johns Hopkins University Press, 1971.

Angel, J. Lawrence. "Paleoecology, Paleodemography and Health." Population, Ecology, and Social Evolution. Steven Polgar, ed. The Hague: Mouton Publishers, 1975, pp. 167-190.

Favazza, Armando R. and Mary Oman. Anthropological and Cross-cultural Themes in Mental Health: An Annotated Bibliography, 1925-1974. University of Missouri Studies LXV. Columbia: University of Missouri Press, 1977.

Grollig, Francis X. and Harold B. Haley, eds. Medical Anthropology. The Hague: Mouton Publishers, 1976.

Landy, David, ed. Culture, Disease, and Healing: Studies in Medical Anthropology. New York: Macmillan Publishing Company, Inc., 1975.

Leslie, Charles, ed. Asian Medical Systems: A Comparative Study. Berkeley: University of California Press, 1976.

Logan, Michael H. and Edward E. Hunt, Jr., eds. Health and the Human Condition: Perspectivies on Medical Anthropology. North Scituate, Massachusetts: Duxbury Press, 1978.

Nag, Moni, ed. Population and Social Organization. The Hague: Mouton Publishers, 1975.

Roche, Alexander F. and Frank Falkner, eds. Nutrition and Malnutrition: Identification and Measurement. Advances in Experimental Medicine and Biology, Volume 49. New York: Plenum Press, 1974.

Westermeyer, Joseph, ed. Anthropology and Mental Health: Setting a New Course. The Hague: Mouton Publishers, 1976.

Part VII.   Demography

Berelson, Bernard, ed. Population Policy in Developed Countries. New York: McGraw-Hill Book Company, 1974.

Glass, D.V. and D.E.C. Eversley, eds. Population in History: Essays in Historical Demography. Chicago: Aldine Publishing Company, 1965.

McCook, Anne S. Health and Population: Research and Policy Issues. Annotated Bibliography, Vol. 3, Number 2. International Program for Population Analysis, Interdisciplinary Communications Program, Smithsonian Institution. Washington: Smithsonian Institution, April 15, 1976.

National Academy of Sciences, National Research Council.
In Search of Population Policy: Views from the Developing
World. Washington: National Academy of Sciences, 1974.

Omran, Abdel R. "Epidemiologic Transition in the U.S.:
The Health Factor in Population Change." Population
Bulletin 32 (2). Washington: Population Reference
Bureau, Inc., 1977.

Preston, Samuel H. "Health Programs and Population Growth."
Population and Development Review 1, 2 (December, 1975):
189-199.

Preston, Samuel H. Mortality Patterns in National
Populations. New York: Academic Press, 1976.

Sheps, Mindel C. and Jeanne Clare Ridley, eds. Public
Health and Population Change: Current Research Issues.
Pittsburgh: University of Pittsburgh Press, 1965.

Taylor, Carl E., Jeanne S. Newman, and Narindar U. Kelly.
"Interactions Between Health and Population." Studies in
Family Planning 7, 4 (April 1976): 94-100.

United Nations. Department of Economic and Social Affairs.
The Determinants and Consequences of Population Trends: New
Summary of Findings on Interaction of Demographic, Economic
and Social Factors. Population Studies, Number 50.
2 Vols. New York: United Nations, 1973.

Part VIII. Economics

Adelman, Irma and Cynthia Taft Morris. Economic Growth and
Social Equity in Developing Countries. Stanford: Stanford
University Press, 1973.

Berg, Alan. The Nutrition Factor: Its Role in National
Development. Washington: The Brookings Institution, 1973.

Brenner, M. Harvey. Estimating the Social Costs of National Economic
Policy: Implications for Mental and Physical Health, and
Criminal Aggression. Achieving the Goals of the Employment
Act of 1946--Thirtieth Anniversary Review, Vol. I,
Paper Number 5. Washington, D.C.: Joint Economic
Committee of the U.S. Congress, 1976.

Culyer, A.J., Jack Wiseman, and Arthur Walker. An Annotated Bibliography of Health Economics. New York: St. Martin's Press, 1977.

Davis, Karen. National Health Insurance: Benefits, Costs, and Consequences. Washington: The Brookings Institution, 1975.

Fuchs, Victor R. Who Shall Live? Health, Economics, and Social Choice. New York: Basic Books, 1974.

Hauser, M.M., ed. The Economics of Medical Care. London: George Allen and Unwin Ltd., 1972.

Health Economics. Geneva: World Health Organization, 1975.

Lave, Lester B. and Eugene P. Seskin. Air Pollution and Human Health. Baltimore: The Johns Hopkins University Press for Resources for the Future, 1977.

Perlman, Marc, ed. The Economics of Health and Medical Care. Proceedings of a conference held by the International Economic Association at Tokyo. New York: Wiley & Sons, 1974.

Sorkin, Alan L. Health Economics. Lexington, Mass.: D.C. Heath, 1975.

Spengler, Joseph J. Population Economics: Selected Essays. Compiled by Robert S. Smith, Frank T. de Vyver, and William R. Allen. Durham, North Carolina: Duke University Press, 1972.

Part IX. History

Bibliography of the History of Medicine. Bethesda, Maryland: National Library of Medicine, annual volumes.

Foucault, Michel. Madness and Civilization: A History of Insanity in the Age of Reason. Richard Howard, translator. New York: Pantheon Books, 1965.

Kass, Edward H. "Infectious Disease and Social Change." The Journal of Infectious Diseases 123 (January 1971): 110-114.

McKeown, Thomas. Medicine in Modern Society: Medical Planning Based on Evaluation of Medical Achievement. New York: Hafner, 1966.

McKinlay, John B. and Sonja M. McKinlay. "The Questionable Effect of Medical Measures on the Decline of Mortality in the United States in the Twentieth Century." Health and Society 55, 3 (Summer 1977): 405-428.

McLachlan, Gordon and Thomas McKeown, eds. Medical History and Medical Care: A Symposium of Perspectives Arranged by the Nuffield Provincial Hospitals Trust and the Josiah Macy, Jr. Foundation. London: Oxford University Press, 1971.

McNeill, William H. Plagues and Peoples. Garden City, New York: Anchor Press, 1976.

Rosen, George. From Medical Police to Social Medicine: Essays on the History of Health Care. New York: Science History Publications, 1974.

Rosen, George. A History of Public Health. New York: MD Publications, Inc., 1958.

Rosen, George. "People, Disease, and Emotion: Some Newer Problems for Research in Medical History." Bulletin of the History of Medicine 41 (1967): 5-23.

Rosenberg, Charles E. The Cholera Years: The United States in 1832, 1849 and 1866. Chicago: University of Chicago Press, 1962.

Rosenkrantz, Barbara G. Public Health and the State: Changing Views in Massachusetts, 1842-1936. Cambridge: Harvard University Press, 1972.

Shyrock, Richard Harrison. Medicine in America: Historical Essays. Baltimore: The Johns Hopkins University Press, 1966.

Stevens, Rosemary. American Medicine and the Public Interest. New Haven: Yale University Press, 1971.

Zinsser, Hans. Rats, Lice and History. Boston: Little Brown, 1935.

Part X. Human Geography

Ackerknecht, E.H. History and Geography of the Most Important Diseases. New York: Hafner, 1965.

DeVise, Pierre. Misused and Misplaced Hospitals and Doctors: A Locational Analysis of the Urban Health Care Crisis. Association of American Geographers, Commission on College Geography. Resource Paper No. 22. Washington: Association of American Geographers, 1973.

Earickson, Robert. The Spatial Behavior of Hospital Patients: A Behavioral Approach to Spatial Interaction in Metropolitan Chicago. University of Chicago, Department of Geography. Research Paper Number 124. Chicago: University of Chicago, 1970.

Girt, John L. "Distance to General Medical Practice and Its Effect on Revealed Ill-Health in a Rural Environment." Canadian Geographer 17, 2 (1973): 154-166.

McGlashan, N.D., ed. Medical Geography: Techniques and Field Studies. London: Methuen & Co., Ltd., 1972.

Pyle, Gerald F. Heart Disease, Cancer and Stroke in Chicago: A Geographical Analysis with Facilities Plans to 1980. University of Chicago, Department of Geography. Research Paper No. 134. Chicago: University of Chicago, 1971.

Pyle, Gerald F. "International Communication and Medical Geography." Social Science and Medicine 11, 14-16 (November 1977): 679-682.

Pyle, Gerald F., ed. "Human Health Problems: Spatial Perspectives." Economic Geography 52, 2 (April 1976): 95-191.

Pyle, Gerald F. and Bruce M. Lauer. "Comparing Spatial Configurations: Hospital Service Areas and Disease Rates." Economic Geography 51, 1 (January 1975): 50-68.

Roboff, Farron Vogel. "The Moving Target: Health Status of Nomadic Peoples." Economic Geography 53, 4 (October 1977): 421-428.

Shannon, Gary W. and G.E. Alan Dever. Health Care
Delivery: Spatial Perspectives. New York: McGraw-
Hill Book Company, 1974.

Smith, Christopher J. The Geography of Mental Health.
Association of American Geographers. Resource Paper
Number 76-4. Washington: Association of American
Geographers, 1977.

Part XI. Philosophy

Gustafson, James M., ed. "Consent and Responsibilities
in Medicine." The Journal of Medicine and Philosophy
2, 4 (December 1977): 305-409.

Medical Research: Statistics and Ethics. Birnbaum
Memorial Symposium. Science 198: 4318 (18 November 1977):
677-705.

Sollitto, Sharmon and Robert M. Veatch, compilers.
Bibliography of Society, Ethics and the Life Sciences,
1976-77. Hastings-on-Hudson, New York: The Hastings
Center, Institute of Society, Ethics and the Life Sciences,
1976.

Taylor, Nancy K., compiler. Bibliography of Society,
Ethics and the Life Sciences, Supplement for 1977-78.
Hastings-on-Hudson, New York: Hastings Center, Institute
of Society, Ethics and the Life Sciences, 1978.

Veatch, Robert M. and Roy Branson, eds. Ethics and Health
Policy . Cambridge: Ballinger Publishing Company, 1976.

Visscher, Maurice B. Ethical Constraints and Imperatives
in Medical Research. Publication number 983 in Bannerstone
division of American lecture series in science and law.
Springfield, Illinois: Charles C. Thomas, 1975.

Walters, LeRoy, ed. Bibliography of Bioethics, Volume 3.
Detroit: Gale Research Company, 1977.

Williams, Preston N., ed. Ethical Issues in Biology and
Medicine. Boston University and American Association for
the Advancement of Science symposium on "The Identity and
Dignity of Man." Cambridge: Schenkman Publishing Co., 1973.

Zaner, Richard M., ed. "Toward a Philosophy of Medicine."
The Journal of Medicine and Philosophy 1, 1 (March 1976):
1-100.

Part XII. Political Science

Cook, Philip and James W. Vaupel, eds. Valuing Lives.
Law and Contemporary Problems 40: 4 (Autumn 1976): 1-305.

Davis, Karen and Cathy Schoen. Health and the War on
Poverty: A Ten-Year Appraisal. Washington: The Brookings
Institution, 1978.

Friedman, Kenneth M. and Stuart H. Rakoff, eds. Toward a
National Health Policy: Public Policy and the Control of
Health Care Costs. Lexington, Massachusetts: Lexington
Books, 1977.

Ginzberg, Eli. The Limits of Health Reform: The Search
for Realism. New York: Basic Books, Inc., 1977.

Ginzberg, Eli, ed. Regionalization and Health Policy.
Washington, D.C.: U.S. Government Printing Office, 1977.

Health Care, Parts I and II. Law and Contemporary Problems
35, 2 (Spring 1970): 229-425 and 35, 4 (Autumn 1970):
667-922.

Heidenheimer, Arnold, Hugh Heclo, and Carolyn Teich Adams.
Comparative Public Policy: The Politics of Social Choice
in Europe and America. New York: St. Martins Press, 1975.

Ilchman, Warren F., et al. Policy Sciences and Population.
Lexington, Massachusetts: Lexington Books, 1975.

Katz, Jay and Alexander Morgan Capron. Catastrophic
Diseases: Who Decides What? A Psychosocial and Legal
Analysis of the Problems Posed by Hemodialysis and Organ
Transplantation. New York: Russell Sage Foundation, 1975.

Levin, Arthur, ed. Health Services: The Local Perspective.
Proceedings of the Academy of Political Science, Vol. 32.
New York: Academy of Political Science, 1977.

Marmor, Theodore R. The Politics of Medicare. Rev. ed.
Chicago: Aldine Publishing Co., 1973.

Medical Progress and the Law. Law and Contemporary Problems 32, 4 (Autumn 1967): 561-750.

Occupational Safety and Health. Law and Contemporary Problems 38, 4 (Summer-Autumn 1974): 583-757.

Strickland, Stephen P. Politics, Science, and Dread Disease: A Short History of United States Medical Research Policy. Cambridge: Harvard University Press, 1972.

Part XIII. Psychiatry

Barrett, J.E., R.M. Rose, and G.L. Klerman, eds. Stress and Mental Disorder. New York: Raven Press, 1979 (forthcoming).

Friedman, Meyer, Ray H. Rosenman and Vernice Carroll. "Changes in the Serum Cholesterol and Blood Clotting Time in Men Subjected to Cyclic Variation of Occupational Stress." Circulation 17 (1958): 852-861.

Gunderson, E.K. Eric and Richard H. Rahe, eds. Life Stress and Illness. Based on contributions to symposium on Life Stress and Illness, sponsored by NATO. Springfield, Illinois: Charles C. Thomas, 1974.

Kasl, Stanislav and Franz Reichsman, eds. Advances in Psychosomatic Medicine, Volume IX. Epidemiologic Studies in Psychosomatic Medicine. Basel: S. Karger, 1977.

Langner, Thomas S. Life Stress and Mental Health. The Midtown Manhattan Study, Volume 2. New York: The Free Press, 1963.

Levi, Lennart, ed. Society, Stress and Disease, Volume 1. The Psychosocial Environment and Psychosomatic Diseases. Proceedings of an international interdisciplinary symposium held in Stockholm, April 1970. London: Oxford University Press, 1971.

Susser, Merwyn W. Community Psychiatry: Epidemiological and Social Themes. New York: Random House, 1968.

Wolff, Harold George. Stress and Disease. 2d ed. Revised and edited by Stewart Wolf and Helen Goodell. Springfield, Illinois: Charles C. Thomas, 1968.

Part XIV. Psychology

Baldwin, Alfred L. Theories of Child Development. New York: Wiley, 1967.

Bush, James W., Robert M. Kaplan, and Charles C. Berry. "Comparison of Methods for Measuring Social Preferences for a Health Status Index." Proceedings of the American Statistical Association, Social Statistics Section, 1977, pp. 682-687.

Cobb, Sidney. "Social Support as a Moderator of Life Stress." Psychosomatic Medicine 38 (1976): 300-314.

Cronbach, Lee J. Essentials of Psychological Testing, 3d Ed. New York: Harper & Row, 1970.

Dohrenwend, Bruce P. and Barbara Snell Dohrenwend. Social Status and Psychological Disorder: A Causal Inquiry. New York: Wiley-Interscience, 1969.

Enelow, A.J. and Henderson, J.B., eds. Conference on Applying Behavioral Science to Cardiovascular Risk. New York: American Heart Association, 1975.

Glass, David C. and Jerome E. Singer, Urban Stress: Experiments on Noise and Social Stressors. New York: Academic Press, 1972.

Hinkle, Lawrence E., Jr. "The Concept of 'Stress' in the Biological and Social Sciences." Science, Medicine and Man 1 (1973): 31-48.

Kaplan, R.M., Bush, J.W., and Berry, C.C. "Health Status: Types of Validity of an Index of Well-Being." Health Services Research 11, 4 (1976): 478-507.

Moss, Gordon E. Illness, Immunity and Social Interaction. New York: Wiley, 1973.

Pomerleau, Ovide , Bass, Frederic and Crown, Victor. "Role of Behavior Modification in Preventive Medicine." New England Journal of Medicine 292 (June 12, 1975): 1277-82.

Williams, R.B. and Gentry, W.D., eds. Behavioral Approaches to Medicine. Cambridge: Ballinger, 1977.

Wolman, Benjamin, et al., eds. Handbook of Clinical
Psychology. New York: McGraw-Hill, 1965.

Part XV. Social Psychology

Becker, Howard S., et al. Boys in White: Student Culture
in Medical School. Chicago: University of Chicago Press,
1961.

Cassel, J. "The Contribution of the Social Environment to
Host Resistance." American Journal of Epidemiology 104, 2
(1976): 107-123.

Hall, Calvin S. and Gardner Lindzey. Theories of Personality,
3d ed. New York: Wiley, 1978.

Kasl, S.V. "The Health Belief Model and Behavior Related
to Chronic Illness". Health Education Monographs 2, 4
(Winter 1974): 433-454.

Levine, Sol and Scotch, Norman A., eds. Social Stress,
Chicago: Aldine, 1970.

Mechanic, David. The Growth of Bureaucratic Medicine: An
Inquiry in the Dynamics of Patient Behavior and the
Organization of Medical Care. New York: Wiley-Inter-
science, 1976.

Meyer, A.J., Maccoby, N., Farquhar, J.W. The Role of
Opinion Leadership in a Cardiovascular Health Education
Campaign. In B.D. Ruben, ed. Communication Yearbook I.
New Brunswick: Transaction Books, 1977.

Rogers, E.M. "Network Analysis of the Diffusion of Family
Planning Innovations." Social Networks: Surveys, Advances
and Commentaries. W. Schramm, D. Lerner, eds. New York:
Academic Press, 1977.

Part XVI. Sociology

Aday, LuAnn and Ronald Andersen. Development of Indices of
Access to Medical Care. Ann Arbor: Health Administration
Press, 1975.

Andersen, Ronald, Joanna Lion, and Odin W. Anderson. Two Decades of Health Services: Social Survey Trends in Use and Expenditure. Cambridge, Mass.: Ballinger Publishing Company, 1976.

Brenner, M. Harvey. Mental Illness and the Economy. Cambridge: Harvard University Press, 1973.

Freeman, Howard E., Sol Levine, and Leo G. Reeder, eds. Handbook of Medical Sociology. 3d ed. Englewood Cliffs, New Jersey: Prentice-Hall, Inc., 1979.

Freidsen, Eliot. Professional Dominance: The Social Structure of Medical Care. New York: Atherton Press, 1970.

Georgopoulos, Basil S. Hospital Organization Research: Review and Source Book. Philadelphia: W.B. Saunders, 1975.

Kosa, John and Irving Kenneth Zola, eds. Poverty and Health: A Sociological Analysis, rev. ed. Commonwealth Fund Book. Cambridge, Mass.: Harvard University Press, 1975.

Krause, Elliott A. Power and Illness: The Political Sociology of Health and Medical Care. New York: Elsevier, 1977.

Mechanic, David. Medical Sociology. 2d ed. New York: Free Press, 1978.

Mechanic, David. Mental Health and Social Policy. Englewood Cliffs, N.J.: Prentice-Hall, Inc., 1969.

Mechanic, David. Politics, Medicine, and Social Science. New York: Wiley-Interscience, 1974.

Susser, M.W. and W. Watson. Sociology in Medicine. 2d ed. London: Oxford University Press, 1971.

Part XVII.   Cross-Disciplinary Research

Barber, Bernard, ed. Medical Ethics and Social Change. The Annals 437 (May 1978): 1-141.

Clarke, Edwin, ed. Modern Methods in the History of Medicine. London: The Athlone Press of the University of London, 1971.

Correa, Hector. Population, Health, Nutrition, and Development: Theory and Planning. Lexington, Mass.: Lexington Books, 1975.

Eisenberg, Leon. "Psychiatry and Society: A Sociobiologic Synthesis." New England Journal of Medicine 296 (21 April, 1977): 903-910.

Engel, George L. "The Need for a New Medical Model: A Challenge for Biomedicine." Science 196: 4286 (8 April, 1977): 129-136.

Fabrega, Horacio, Jr. Disease and Social Behavior: An Interdisciplinary Perspective. Cambridge, Mass.: The MIT Press, 1974.

Galdston, Iago, ed. The Interface Between Psychiatry and Anthropology. New York: Brunner/Mazel, Publishers, 1971.

Glass, David V. and Roger Revelle, eds. Population and Social Change. Conference proceedings sponsored by Harvard Center for Population Studies and the American Academy of Arts and Sciences. London: Edward Arnold, 1972.

Goldscheider, Calvin. Population, Modernization, and Social Structure. Boston: Little, Brown and Company, 1971.

Insel, Paul M. and Rudolph H. Moos, eds. Health and the Social Environment. Lexington, Mass.: Lexington Books, 1974.

Leslie, Charles, ed. Special Issue: Theoretical Foundations for the Comparative Study of Medical Systems. Social Science and Medicine 12: 2B (April 1978): 65-138.

McKeown, Thomas. The Modern Rise of Population. New York: Academic Press, 1976.

Redlich, F.C., ed. "Concepts of Health and Disease." The Journal of Medicine and Philosophy 1, 3 (September 1976): 201-280.

Reining, Priscilla and Irene Tinker, eds. Population: Dynamics, Ethics and Policy. Washington: American Association for the Advancement of Science, 1975.

Rosen, George. "Health, History and the Social Sciences." Social Science and Medicine 7 (April 1973): 233-248.

Part XVIII.   Social Epidemiological Studies That Include
Health Care

Bromet, Evelyn et al.   "Posttreatment Functioning of Alcoholic
Patients: Its Relation to Program Participation." Journal
of Counseling and Clinical Psychology 45 (1977): 829-842.

Croog, Sydney H. and Sol Levine. The Heart Patient Recovers:
Social and Psychological Factors. New York: Human Sciences
Press, 1977.

Meyer, Henry H. and Edgar F. Borgatta. An Experiment in Mental Patient Rehabilitation. New York: Russell Sage Foundation, 1959.

Riedel, Donald C., Gary L. Tischler, and Jerome K. Myers, eds.
Patient Care Evaluation in Mental Health Programs. Cambridge,
Mass.: Ballinger Publishing Co., 1974.

Suchman, Edward A. "A Model for Research and Evaluation on
Rehabilitation." In Marvin B. Sussman, ed., Sociology and
Rehabilitation. Washington: American Sociological Associ-
ation, 1965.

Part 1

Social, Structural and Demographic Factors

Introduction: Part 1

The field of health is a field in crisis and transition. Recent research findings have raised serious questions regarding the validity of traditional health theory, and are forcing a critical re-examination of the assumptions on which the theory is based and the conceptual approach to which it has given rise. Indeed, it is probably not too much to say that the field is experiencing a paradigm shift (Kuhn, 1970), a process that will ultimately give rise to a radical restructuring of health theory and a fundamental reorientation of the way health problems are defined and policies are conceptualized.

The Traditional Health Paradigm

The traditional health paradigm is based on the assumption that health and mortality levels are primarily a function of the interaction between the individual and the physical environment, including physical contact with other, diseased individuals. Another fundamental assumption is that the delivery of modern (i.e., Western) medical technology and associated services has been primarily responsible for observed declines in mortality and broad improvements in national and international health trends and levels.

These basic assumptions have given rise to particular definitions of health problems and issues; they have also generated two fundamental strategies for improving health levels among human populations. The first is the curative, or clinical, approach, which relies on medical technology and services to relieve disease symptoms and/or to cure diseases after they have been contracted. This approach is clinic- and hospital-based, and consumes the vast bulk of health sector effort in all save a few nations today (World Bank, 1975). The second strategy is the public health, or preventive, approach, which utilizes medical technology to mediate between the individual and the physical environment in ways that will lessen the probability of contracting diseases. Mediation may take the form of environmental modification, as in protecting water supplies and spraying mosquitos; or modification of the individual through such tactics as vaccination, and attitude, value, and behavior change through health education (Brown and Margo, 1978). Programs of training health personnel have therefore focused primarily on the technical and technological aspects of medicine, and their efficient delivery, as well as techniques of "motivation," or behavior modification.

It is notable that none of these conventional strategies attempts to influence health levels by modifying the social, human-created environment in which the individual lives and must act. That is, attempts to influence health levels have taken place within the confines of "the system," which is taken as given. The result is strategies of change that are of a first order nature,[1] in that they do not affect the established system itself (Warzlawick, et al., 1974). The social environment itself is not considered to be variable or instrumental, or even problematic, and perhaps in need of second order change as a condition necessary to effect widespread improvements in health trends and levels.

Given these basic assumptions and strategies, it is unsurprising that the adoption and diffusion of innovations[2] has been the conceptual approach that has dictated health research foci and priorities, conclusions drawn from research findings, and policy recommendations for some four decades (Rogers, 1962). Despite the fact that the "early adopters" of modern medical technology and services are consistently characterized by higher income and education, and by greater physical and material security, these are rarely viewed as structural features. Indeed, the key factors limiting the diffusion of modern health levels are assumed to be the conservative values and fatalistic attitudes of the poor and uneducated segments of society. This approach also assumes that modern health behavior spreads from more innovative to less innovative individuals through a "multiplier effect." The practical effect of this approach is to justify the concentration of available resources and services among the more advantaged groups and urban enclaves, while relying on an indirect, or "trickle down," effect to reach the poor and disadvantaged.[3]

The Emergent Paradigm

Within the past few years, however, a new paradigm has emerged that is challenging the conventional paradigm for dominance among the scientific community. The emergent paradigm is based on research relevant to the field of health that has illuminated the relationship between structural factors and the health processes. Such research has shown that available evidence does not support the proposition that observed mortality declines are attributable to the diffusion of medical technology and services. Indeed, the analysis of disease trends makes it apparent that "the specifically medical treatment of people is nowhere and never significantly related to a decline in the compound disease burden or to a rise in life expectancy" (Illich, 1975: 18).

The implication is not that modern medicine has been without impact; rather, the impact of modern medicine on mortality trends and levels has been vastly overrated. As one reviewer notes:

> Some modern techniques, often developed with the contribution of doctors, and optimally effective when they become part of the environment or are applied by the general public, have determined changes in health, but to a lesser degree. Into this category belong contraceptives and such non-medical health measures as the treatment of water or excrement, the use of soap and scissors by midwives, the smallpox vaccination of infants, and a few antibacterials and insecticides (Illich, 1975: 18).

In fact, particular curative and preventive measures served only to accelerate slightly the substantial declines in mortality already well under way before either the germ theory or specific causes of disease received wide acceptance (Powles, 1973). The historical epidemiological and sociological evidence indicates that improvements in such socioeconomic conditions as education, nutrition, housing, sanitation, and working conditions combined to bring about mortality reductions and increased life expectancies--not medical science and medical care (Powles, 1973). Of particular importance among the causes of mortality reductions and increased life expectancies is improved nutritional status. It is evident that acute, infectious, and epidemic diseases thrive in populations where host-resistance has been weakened by material deprivation. In areas where malnutrition is widespread, infectious diseases are the major causes of death among children under five years of age (Bodenheimer, 1972). Moreover, it has been demonstrated that diarrhea and respiratory infections are more frequent, longer-lasting, and cause more deaths in poor, malnourished populations regardless of how much or how little medical care is available (Scrimshaw et al., 1968). Control of these diseases has occurred largely through improvements in the production and, particularly, distribution of food (Goldscheider, 1971).

Education also appears to be a major factor influencing mortality and life expectancy in both developed and underdeveloped countries. With regard to socioeconomic differentials in mortality in the United States, education has been shown to be the single most powerful explanatory variable; it is even more important than income (Kitagawa and Hauser, 1973: 23). In underdeveloped countries, observed mortality declines are better explained by improved levels of education than by either economic growth rates or medical inputs (Preston, 1976). Indeed, educational levels appear to determine whether or not public health inputs will be effective in reducing disease levels. For example, it has been found that the use of privies by populations lacking education has little or no effect on the prevalence of infectious diseases, and at times has even had a negative impact (Scrimshaw et al., 1968; Van Zijl, 1966). Exactly how education influences mortality and life expectancy is not yet well-understood; but it is known that the most effective preventive health measures are those applied at the individual level on a daily basis (e.g., personal hygiene, treatment of food, storage and use of water, etc.). Since the results of such preventive health measures do not lend themselves to empirical verification (i.e., they are "non-events"), their continued and effective application apparently requires an understanding at the conceptual level by the individual applying the measure (Foster, 1976).

Although improved levels of nutrition and education may rank first among the socioeconomic factors responsible for declining mortality, others are not far behind in importance: improved levels of personal income and employment also contribute to host improvement and, thus, to reductions in mortality and increased life expectancies (Dubos, 1976). But a major point to be noted is that observed levels of income, education, socioeconomic class, and, therefore, nutritional and mortality levels, are themselves determined not by the physical environment but by the political and economic system in which they are embedded. This situation is not often well-understood, for it tends to be obscured by the traditional, and continuing, focus of health professionals upon the relationship between the individual and the physical environment (Brown and Margo, 1978).

Societal attempts to exert control over the physical environment have led to the development of sociopolitical and economic systems designed to assist individual members better to cope with that environment through the distribution of available knowledge and technology (Goldscheider, 1971). Over time, these socially designed systems have become more important than the physical environment to individual surviv- al because they control the distribution of and access to those very factors that now determine mortality levels. Indeed,

> ...there has been a major shift from those sources of human stress stemming from the physical environ- ment to those stemming from the social environment. It is interesting to note that this social environ- ment is precisely the one designed by man himself in order to better control physical environmental problems.... Even in advanced industrialized soci- eties, trends in the infant mortality rate are still largely dependent on fluctuations in the national economy. This is true not only for the United States, but of countries such as England, and parti- cularly Sweden, which are well-known for their com- plete and rigorous health coverage (Brenner, 1976).[4]

To be sure, the physical environment still exacts a certain toll through such incidents as earthquakes, tidal waves, floods, and long-term climatic changes. Nevertheless, the socioeconomic systems created by and for people constitute, to all intents and purposes, the human individual's "natural" environment.

The importance to mortality and life expectancies of the socially designed environment cannot be overemphasized. The institutions created by and established within society to mediate between the individual and the physical environment now play central roles in determining societal mortality rates by the manner in which they distribute income, educa- tion, food, technology, and employment/unemployment. In most societies, these factors are distributed differentially among groups and individuals according to their place in the socio- economic stratification system. And "...differences in socioeconomic status are responsible for differences in mor- tality" (Kitagawa and Hauser, 1973: 20).

It must be emphasized that these research findings do not represent merely an increment to what is already known about the health process, for they demonstrate that institu- tional factors are more powerful determinants of demographic trends and levels than such assumed barriers to technological

adoption and diffusion as fatalism, illiteracy, conservative
values and traditional modes of behavior, and limited media
exposure. Instead, this research suggests that a fundamental
reconstruction of prior theory and a reinterpretation of prior
fact in light of a new theory are necessary.

The research findings mentioned above are only a sampling of the host that are inexplicable by traditional health
theory and are anomalous within the conventional health paradigm. For these reasons, a new theory of health has emerged
that is based on these research findings and attempts to
account for them within a new paradigm. The emergent paradigm maintains that mortality and health trends and levels
are primarily functions of the social, political, and economic context within which the individual lives and must act.
Individual characteristics are therefore seen as less important determinants of health and mortality than social stratification within society. Indeed, it asserts that the differential distribution of resources, goods, and services
within society is the primary determinant of differential
mortality and morbidity levels observed to exist between
social groups and classes. The major postulate of this paradigm is: to the degree that all segments of society share
equitably in the benefits of development, mortality and morbidity will decline. This paradigm views those political and
economic institutions that control the distribution of available resources as posing both the greatest threats to and
hopes for improved levels of mortality and increased life
expectancies around the world. For, indeed, these institutions determine who shall live and who shall die.

The research papers presented in this volume shed new
light on both the conventional and emergent paradigms.
Nathan Keyfitz addresses the problems of measuring mortality
that stem from the conventional mode of treating populations
as if they were homogeneous instead of heterogeneous. It is
clear, as Keyfitz notes, that "whatever the hazard, some
people are more subject to it than others." He concludes
that the diminishing returns to conventional health approaches may be due to the fact that "the entities under attack are not the appropriate ones." Keyfitz brings particular aspects of demographic theory to bear on this problem in
his attempt to define a new phase of mortality analysis.

Harvey Brenner, in an extension of some of his earlier,
seminal research, presents the results of a careful examination of the relationship between health trends and fluctuations in rates of economic growth. He finds that "economic
instability," whether it be measured in terms of rising unemployment or sharply accelerating economic growth, results

in increased mortality rates among affected populations. In this investigation, Brenner attempts to delineate both the beneficial and detrimental aspects of economic growth as they affect human populations. An important outcome of this study is an equation, presented here for the first time, by which mortality trends in human populations can be statistically explained. This equation includes secular and short-term trends in real per-capita income and its distribution, unemployment rates, educational levels, and public welfare expenditures.

Jude Thomas May, Katherine Parry, Mary Durham, and Peter New illustrate, in their case-study analysis of the planning and implementation of OEO-funded neighborhood health centers, how political and economic institutions can provide barriers to innovation in the delivery of health care to the disadvantaged sectors of society. In their paper, they show how the process of bureaucratization can be shifted from goal-oriented functions to system-maintenance functions due to such sociopolitical and economic forces as limitation of program resources and the need for rapid professional legitimation. They conclude from their findings that the existing system must, once again, assume substantial responsibility for the fact that low-income populations are limited in their access to adequate health services.

Notes

1. First order change is incremental in nature, and does not affect the basic structural properties of a system. Second order change is fundamental in nature, and transforms the basic structure of the system itself. See P. Watzlawick, J. Weakland, and R. Fisch. Change; Principles of Problem Formation and Problem Resolution. New York: W.W. Norton and Co., 1974.

2. For a summary of early diffusionist theory and research, and for the most clearly articulated and seminal source of influence in the field, see E. Rogers. Diffusion of Innovations. New York: Free Press, 1962.

3. For a recent, detailed review and critique of the diffusion of innovations approach, see E. Saint and E.W. Coward. "Agriculture and Behavioral Science: Emerging Orientations." Science 197, 19 (August 1977): 733-737.

4. See M.H. Brenner, "Mortality, Social Stress, and the Modern Economy: Experience of the United States, Britain, and Sweden, 1900-1970," paper presented at the Annual Meeting of the American Association for the Advancement of

Science, Boston, February 21, 1976, pp. 13-14; for a more general discussion, see also pp. 1-5.

References

Bodenheimer, T.S.   "The Political Economy of Malnutrition: Generalization from Two Central American Case Studies." Archivos Latino-Americanos de Nutricion 22 (1972): 495-505.

Brenner, M.H.   "Mortality, Social Stress, and the Modern Economy: Experience of the United States, Britain, and Sweden, 1900-1970." Paper presented at the Annual Meeting of the American Association for the Advancement of Science, Boston, February 21, 1976.

Brown, E.R. and G.E. Margo.   "Health Education: Can the Reformers Be Reformed?" International Journal of Health Services 8, 1 (1978): 3-26.

Dubos, R. Man Adapting. New Haven, Conn.: Yale University Press, 1967.

Foster, G.M.   "Medical Anthropology and International Health Planning." Medical Anthropology Newsletter 7, 3 (May 1976): 14

Goldscheider, C.   "The Mortality Revolution." In Population, Modernization, and Social Structure. Boston: Little, Brown and Co., 1971.

Illich, I. Medical Nemesis; the Expropriation of Health. London: Marion Boyars, 1975.

Kitagawa, E.M. and P.M. Hauser. Differential Mortality in the United States: A Study in Socioeconomic Epidemiology. Cambridge: Harvard University Press, 1973.

Kuhn, T. The Structure of Scientific Revolutions (2nd ed.). Chicago: University of Chicago Press, 1970.

Powles, J.   "On the Limitations of Modern Medicine." Science, Medicine and Man 1 (1973): 1-30.

Preston, S.H.   "Determinants of Mortality Declines in Less-Developed Countries, 1940-1970." Paper presented at the Annual Meeting of the American Association for the Advancement of Science, Boston, February 21, 1976.

Rogers, E. Diffusion of Innovations. New York: Free Press, 1962.

Saint, E. and E.W. Coward. "Agriculture and Behavioral Science: Emerging Orientations." Science 197, 19 (August 1977): 733-737.

Scrimshaw, N.S., C.E. Taylor, and J.E. Gordon. Interaction of Nutrition and Infection. Geneva: World Health Organization, 1968.

Van Zijl, W.J. "Studies on Diarrhoeal Diseases in Seven Countries by the WHO Diarrhoeal Diseases Advisory Team." Bulletin of The World Health Organization 35, 2 (1966): 249-261

Watzlawick, P., J. Weakland, and R. Fisch. Change; Principles of Problem Formation and Problem Resolution. New York: W.W. Norton and Co., 1974.

World Bank. Assault on World Poverty; Problems of Rural Development, Education, and Health. Baltimore: Johns Hopkins University Press, 1975.

1. Demographic Methods and Their Application in the Social and Health Sciences

Physicians deal with individual patients. There is no way of treating sick people en masse; all therapeutic procedures that I know of deal with them one by one. The diagnosis of sickness is by categories suited to the therapeutic procedures available.

The community aspects of disease, arising from environmental hazards of many kinds, gave rise to collective "therapy" that combined preventive medicine and engineering in a new field of public health. Since those early beginnings, communities and community life have become more complex and the health problems that they throw up correspondingly complex. Public health has come to embrace elements of biological, physical, and social science.

Within public health, epidemiology investigates diseases of unknown etiology; it uses statistical methods to track diseases back to their (collective or individual) causes. Some striking relations show up in the statistical analysis that would never be observed in patients considered one by one. Brian MacMahon has recently found that women who have had at least one child are less likely to fall victim to breast cancer than women who have had no children. Epidemiologists and biostatisticians make life tables for groups who have been treated with competing therapies, and compare survivorships. Once the etiology of a disease and its treatment are thoroughly understood, many of the statistical techniques of the epidemiologists are no longer needed, and they go on to other problems; there is no danger of their running out of problems.

Demographers are not directly concerned with health as such, but rather with the factors that govern the increase and decline of populations. Their primary interest is the processes of birth, death, and migration; they are concerned with characteristics of populations, including age, sex, and marital status; and spatial, occupational, and other distributions. They examine average life cycles of individuals and of families. Though cause of death is one of their major interests, their focus is not so much health and disease as it is population change. They obtain data from vital registrations of birth and death as well as from censuses; with the advent of sampling techniques and organizations, surveys, especially of fertility, have permitted them to collect their own data rather than having to depend on data collected for other purposes.

Thus demography includes a set of problems (how populations increase and decrease), various techniques (life tables, the renewal equation), the sources of data (vital registrations, censuses). There are many ways in which this collection of problems, methods, and data interact with public health, and I will be forgiven for not attempting to treat all of them.

What I will do is contrast the progress of medicine in recent decades with its small demographic effect. In the treatment and care of the individual patient, the capacity, both qualitative and quantitative, has been expanding without intermission; every year new drugs are discovered, new surgical procedures are devised, new facts are uncovered in the relation of behavior (e.g., smoking) to mortality. Meanwhile, nothing is ever lost of effective old ways of treatment. The steadily increasing overall effectiveness of medicine that results is not only in keeping people alive but in making the procedures more efficient and more comfortable, though this latter aspect will be disregarded here. The demographer does not differentiate as long as the body is warm.

Insofar as physicians or others think of cases collectively, they are likely to do so in terms of rates. These rates may be the fraction that survive a surgical procedure; the fraction of diagnosed cancer cases that die within a year; or the death rate among those sustaining a certain kind of brain injury. In any of these, a rate twice as high is twice as bad.

An alternative way of thinking of these questions, for which I shall present a case, is in terms of the mean time to death. As the expectation of life, this is a well-known parameter, perhaps the most often used measure of health to be found in the demographic literature. We speak of the expectation of life as being about 30 years in 18th century Europe; of its gradual rise through the 19th and 20th

centuries to over 70 years; and of its much quicker rise
since World War II among many peoples of Asia to 60 or more.
In many Latin American countries, the expectation of life
has been going up at one year per year; that can continue
for only a short time, but it shows the rapidity of progress.

Is there really any difference between citing a figure
that shows a decline in the death rate and one that shows an
increase in the expectation of life? After all, it can be
shown by the most rigorous mathematics that, in a group
where the death rate is μ , the expected time to death will
be $1/\mu$. But that is on the assumption of homogeneity: supposing every individual separately is subject to the same
risk μ . We will find that where the population is heterogeneous, with some individuals subject to a different risk
from others, the expectation of life can be very far from
the reciprocal of the death rate.

This is an old story for heterogeneity with respect to
age and sex. The exigencies of the insurance business
brought the point painfully to the attention of actuaries in
18th century England. The death rate in a certain community
may be 0.02, but if one offers to insure people at a premium
of $20 per thousand irrespective of age, the clientele of
the insurance company will consist of old people, and the
company will quickly go bankrupt. This is a kind of heterogeneity that everyone knows about, and it has been thoroughly taken into account during the past two centuries. The
same is true of the difference between the sexes; female
annuitants, as the companies found at an early stage, live
longer than male annuitants, and they have to be charged
correspondingly higher rates.

But the companies were discouraged from discriminating
according to other kinds of heterogeneity, for insurance
depends on the averaging of risks. If any kind of examination could reveal at exactly what age an individual would
die, insurance could not exist. Actuarial science, and
hence demography, which obtained some of its techniques from
actuarial science, treat populations as homogeneous within
age and sex groups.

Yet, assuming homogeneity gives grossly wrong results
in assessing the benefit of a medical improvement. Ultimately, no one cares about lowering death rates; what they
want is increased expectation of life. Which measure is
used greatly affects the conclusions about the benefit obtained from a medical improvement. What seems like an important gain when one assumes homogeneity can become small
when underlying heterogeneity in the population is recognized.

Hence, a preferred way of surveying American mortality trends, using the officially calculated expectation of life $\overset{o}{e}_0$, shows that:

1) Male expectation is less than female, and the difference increases over time.

2) There is convergence between whites and all others, but with some gap still remaining in 1975.

3) There is much more improvement in $\overset{o}{e}_0$ than in $\overset{o}{e}_{60}$.

4) For most groups, the increase during the course of this century has been about one-third of a year of life per year of time.

5) There has been great unevenness in improvement among decades, with the largest improvement in the 1930's and the smallest in the 1960's.

These trends and differences are not easily explained in terms of the effectiveness of medical knowledge and access to it. The greatest improvement was shown in the 1930's, the smallest in the 1960's; though antibiotics came into use in the 1930's, there was also economic depression and high unemployment that must have made access to good medicine more difficult for some strata of the population. On the other hand, the 1960's were far and away the most prosperous decade in American history by whatever measure one applies, and the decade was not lacking in medical progress; but the increase in life expectation was trifling.

Again, the application of medicine to older people has been steadily expanding to ever broader social strata, but little increase in life expectation has resulted. Moreover there can be no serious contention that men have had less access to medicine than women, but the improvement for women has been far greater than for men.

Especially striking is the rather small variation in the expectation of life. White females show about 8 years more than white males in 1975, an excess of 12 percent. Yet the probability that a white female lives to age 85 is 0.35, while the probability that a white male lives to that age is 0.16, less than half as much. At particular ages, moreover, the death rates for males are as much as twice those for females. Indexes weighting the rates for the several ages show male mortality to be 50 to 90 percent higher than female. Thus, the most appropiate measure of mortality improvement, expectation of life, seems to show very small differences among groups and over time as compared with age-specific death rates.

The reason why the differences in $\overset{o}{e}_0$ are small is that little further improvement in mortality is possible at younger ages. Fully 88 percent of white females and 78 percent of white males live to age 60. At the beginning of the century, fewer than half of all children born lived to age 60. At one time, the curve of survivorship sloped downward through life; in recent decades it has moved more and more towards the horizontal, until about age 70, where it takes a sharp fall.

An application of differential calculus provides a measure of this. Multiply all the age-specific death rates $\mu(x)$ by $1 + \delta$; this takes the survivorship to the power $\ell^{1+\delta}(x)$, and the expectation is $\overset{o}{e}_0 = \int_0^\omega \ell^{1+\delta}(x)\,dx$. Now differentiate this with respect to δ, to obtain at $\delta = 0$ the derivative

$$\frac{d\overset{o}{e}_0}{d\delta} = -H\overset{o}{e}_0 ,$$

where H is minus the logarithm of the probability of surviving, averaged over all ages with the numbers surviving as the weights:

$$H = -\frac{\int_0^\omega \ell(x)\ln\,\ell(x)\,dx}{\int_0^\omega \ell(x)\,dx} .$$

This shows, by an easy application of differential calculus, that a 1 percent decrease in all age-specific death rates corresponds to an increase in $\overset{o}{e}_0$, not of 1 percent, but of H percent. At the beginning of the century, H was about 0.40; today it is about 0.20 for males, 0.16 for females.

Now to proceed to particular causes of death. Consider the following way of answering the question, "How much increase in the expectation of life would result from the elimination of cancer?" The expectation of life for males in 1975 is 69 years, so the death rate in the stationary condition would be 1/69. Cancer deaths are 0.17 of all deaths, so their elimination ought to reduce the death rate by

Table 1. Percent increase in expectation of life at birth associated with one-percent drop in age-cause-specific mortality, United States males, 1964.

Causes of Death	If other causes remain the same in total	If other causes remain the same age by age
Respiratory tuberculosis	0.0055	0.0012
Other infectious and parasitic	0.0053	0.0018
Neoplasms	0.1570	0.0302
Cardiovascular renal	0.5688	0.0840
Influenza, pneumonia, bronchitis	0.0368	0.0078
Diarrheal	0.0033	0.0012
Certain degenerative	0.0414	0.0090
Certain diseases of infancy	0.0167	0.0170
Motor vehicle	0.0266	0.0129
Other violence	0.0503	0.0192
Other and unknown	0.0883	0.0232
Total	1.0000	0.2073

Source: Calculated from data in Samuel H. Preston, N. Keyfitz, and R. Schoen, Causes of Death: Life Tables for National Populations (New York: Seminar Press, 1972).

17 percent; the death rate would become 83 percent of 1/69 or 0.01203. Hence, the expectation of life would be the reciprocal of this, or 83 years. We would have added 83 - 69 = 14 years by eliminating cancer.

This calculation is mostly correct. If we disregard population growth, which is small anyway, it is true that the death rate is the reciprocal of the expectation of life, and our using this fact twice is justified. It is also true that, if the cancer deaths were eliminated and nothing else changed, then the death rate would go down by the 17 percent we used, the fraction of deaths that are due to cancer.

What is incorrect in the calculation is supposing everything else would be the same. It is self-contradictory to assume that cancer is eliminated and that death rates from other causes remain the same. For, with the elimination of cancer and with people living to a somewhat older age, the deaths due to other ailments would increase. People would move into the ages at which they would be subject to heart disease and other degenerative causes of death. If this is taken into account, holding constant not the total deaths from other causes but age-specific rates, the improvement is brought down from 17 percent to a very much smaller amount: to about 2 years, given the base expectation of 69 years, or only 3 percent.

Let us go through this calculation again, now thinking not of eradication of cancer but of a 1 percent reduction in cancer deaths. By the same method as above, but multiplying age-specific cancer deaths $\mu^{(i)}(x)$ by $1 + \delta$ and then differentiating $\overset{o}{e}_0$ with respect to δ, we find

$$\frac{d\overset{o}{e}_0}{d\delta} = -H^{(i)} \overset{o}{e}_0 \ ,$$

where $H^{(i)}$ is the same as H but having $\ln \ell^{(i)}(x)$ instead of $\ln \ell(x)$. The values of $H^{(i)}$ for 12 main causes are shown in Table 1. Thus, neoplasms show at 0.0302; this means that a drop of 1 percent in cancer deaths would raise $\overset{o}{e}_0$ by 0.030 percent if other causes remain the same age by age. But if other causes remained the same in total, $\overset{o}{e}_0$ would go up by 0.157 percent.

Our next question is to find how a decline in deaths from the $\underline{i}$th cause $\mu^{(i)}(x)$ affects the overall death rate from the $\underline{j}$th cause $d^{(j)}$. When the age-specific death rates

due to cancer go down, relatively more people will die of
heart disease. Let us ascertain how many more, assuming
that age-specific rates for heart disease do not change, so
that the increase will be due only to the change in the age
distribution of the population arising from the fall in cancer deaths. We need an expression for the increase in the
crude rate for heart disease when there is a fall in the
age-specific rates for cancer.

In general notation, suppose that the deaths from the
ith cause change by a uniform fraction δ at all ages,
which is to say that from being $\mu^{(i)}(x)$ they go to
$\mu^{(i)}(x)(1 + \delta)$. The probability of surviving accordingly
changes from $\ell(x)$ to $\ell(x)\ell^{(i)\delta}(x)$, where $\ell^{(i)}(x)$ is the
chance of surviving to age x in the face of only the ith
cause. Similar notation applies to the jth cause. The
crude death rate for the jth cause in the original stationary condition is

$$d^{(j)} = \int_0^\omega \ell(x)\mu^{(j)}(x)\,dx/\overset{o}{e}_0 ,$$

and in the new condition is

$$d^{(j)*} = \int_0^\omega \ell(x)\ell^{(i)\delta}(x)\mu^{(j)}(x)\,dx/\overset{o}{e}_0^* ,$$

or, to a linear approximation,

$$d^{(j)*} = d^{(j)} + \frac{[\int_0^\omega \ell(x)\ln\ell^{(i)}(x)\mu^{(j)}(x)\,dx]\delta}{\overset{o}{e}_0} .$$

So much for the effect of continuance of the age-specific rates. We now attempt to see what the result would be
of supposing some kind of linkage among the several causes.

The categories of cause of death that are used in vital
statistics are elaborations of those developed for purposes
of medical diagnosis. Since the purpose of diagnosis is
treatment, the causal system that physicians use has evolved
to correspond to the methods successful in treating individual patients. It is important to know whether a patient is
suffering from cancer of one site rather than another if
local treatment is to be applied. But if a general way of

preventing the multiplication of cancerous cells anywhere in the body were to be found, then diagnosis by site would be less important. More broadly yet, if cancer and heart disease are manifestations of a deterioration of the process by which normal cells reproduce, say through errors in copying the DNA code, then diagnosis even according to the gross categories of cancer, heart disease, etc., would become unimportant.

In the present state of knowledge, no one can prove that there are certain underlying causes of the several degenerative diseases, or perhaps a single cause for all; but the possibility is suggested by the fact that they tend to strike at similar ages. Moreover, many of those who die of one of these causes are listed as suffering from others; multiple causes of death are far too frequent to permit the assumption that the several presently designated causes are wholly independent.

It is out of order to suggest that the presently designated causes be disregarded as long as current therapies are the best we have. The present argument does not concern either therapy or the tabulation of vital statistics as now performed. But it does concern the direction of research.

In accord with this, we suppose some elementary uncorrelated factors of mortality, still functions of age, say $\nu^{(i)}(x)$; and take it that the observed death rates $\mu^{(i)}(x)$ are linear combinations of these. Then the vector of the $\mu^{(i)}(x)$ can be expressed as

$$\mu^{(i)}(x) = a_{i1}\nu^{(1)}(x) \ldots a_{in}\nu^{(n)}(x) \ , \ i = 1, 2, \ldots, m,$$

or in matrix form,

$$\mu(x) = A \, \nu(x),$$

where $\mu(x)$ is 1xm, $\nu(x)$ is 1xn, both vertical vectors.

We can calculate the $\ell^{(i)}(x)$ as a column vector from

$$\begin{bmatrix} \ln \ell^{(1)}(x) \\ \ln \ell^{(2)}(x) \\ \cdot \\ \cdot \\ \cdot \\ \ln \ell^{(m)}(x) \end{bmatrix} = -A \int_{0}^{\omega} \nu(a)\,da,$$

then go on to find the expectation of life $\overset{o}{e}_0$ as a function of the $\nu^{(i)}(x)$, using the method developed by Volterra for such a purpose.

All this is mere formalism unless some way can be found to calculate the a's and the ν's. This may be possible by the methods of factor analysis, using either longitudinal or cross-sectional data.

Rene Dubos has illuminating observations on our notion that each disease has a specific cause. The notion is only about 100 years old. Prior to that, the Hippocratean idea prevailed: disease was due to lack of harmony between the sick person and his environment, or among the four humors. For the Chinese, disease was the upsetting of the proper balance between the yin and the yang.

Harmony and balance lost their place in medicine in the latter part of the 19th century, when Pasteur and Koch showed by laboratory experiments that disease could be produced at will by introducing a single specific factor, a virulent microorganism, into a healthy animal.

From the field of infection, the doctrine of specific etiology spread to other areas of medicine. A large variety of well-defined disease states could be produced experimentally by recreating in the body specific biochemical or physiological lesions (Dubos, 1959: 103). By analogy to smallpox, we call cancer a disease and assume there is some specific cause, and all we have to do is find the equivalent of an antibiotic for a cure. But suppose that cancer is the outcome of a constellation of circumstances rather than of any one factor. Even in diseases caused by germs, this is demonstrably so. Much of the European population in the 19th century carried tuberculosis germs, but only a fraction showed the disease. Part of the etiology had to be sought in the relation of the person to his environment.

Even effective therapies do not constitute evidence for the doctrine of specific etiology, says Dubos. There are many cases where a disease can be controlled by several unrelated procedures. "The most that can be said (of cholera) is that once the vidrios have become established in the intestinal tract, some other factor can convert the infection into a disease." (Dubos, 1959: 108)

But the most crushing evidence that the germs are not the disease is the decline of infectious diseases, which took place very early. Mortality from tuberculosis has been

falling steadily since the middle of the 19th century in
Europe and America, prior to drug therapy and vaccination.
"The campaign for pure food, pure water, and pure air" had
much to do with the conquest of epidemic disease (Dubos,
1959: 151).

We cannot cite Rene Dubos without giving equal time to
the opposition. In one aspect, that is represented by Lewis
Thomas, president of the Memorial Sloan-Kettering Cancer
Center in New York. He agrees that germs alone do not cause
disease: healthy people can contain germs of many potentially fatal diseases, but the symbiosis is harmless. In respect
to meningitis, the meningococcus "has nothing to gain ...
from getting into the bloodstream and infecting the central
nervous system. The organism gets along fine by living in
the nasal and throat mucosa of the host. It must be even
more of a catastrophe for a meningococcus to catch a man
than for a man to catch a meningococcus." (Bernstein, 1978:
40) Thus, visible disease is a kind of accident that dis-
turbs a previously innocuous man-parasite relation.

Nonetheless, there is often one element that triggers
the disease and that can be called its cause. At one time,
we thought that tuberculosis was an environmental disease.
"We had theories about air--bad air, moist air, night air--
being bad for it. All kinds of diet were cooked up to influence it one way or the other... Bed rest... Go to Arizona....
But once we had a technology that would get rid of the tuber-
cle bacillus, that was it.... Every disease that we do know
about ... turns out to be a disease in which there is one
central mechanism.... In the case of pneumonia it is the
pneumococcus, ... in pellagra it is a single vitamin deficiency." (Bernstein, 1978: 44) There is no reason to think
any differently about the diseases that remain: cancer,
coronary occlusion, stroke, and the kind of kidney disease
that develops into chronic kidney failure.

The expectation of life is taken here as the criterion
for measuring the effect of a health improvement. In a
homogeneous population, where everyone is subject to the
same risk, the reduction in the rate and the increase of the
expectation of life are the same thing, and no one can object
to using either one as the criterion. But in a heterogeneous
population, a value judgment in the selection of the criterion is inescapable. A man of 30 could well say that he
is not especially interested in increase of expectation at
age zero, but only in expectation at age 30. Or that, insofar as a person has heard that he stands in special danger
from cancer, he will favor research on cancer rather than on
heart disease. The most that one can say for the use of

expectation of life at age zero is that it includes mortality at all ages and is not grossly biased towards any one group.

Joel E. Cohen (1975) takes the argument one stage farther. He goes on to find the lifetime earnings of the individuals whose lives would be saved by a medical innovation, and thus is able to establish a dollar value for the benefit. For example, he finds $20 billion as the lower bound of the benefit from eliminating kidney and related diseases in the United States. In the present paper, we stop with the expectation of life rather than earnings as the ultimate criterion.

The decision on what direction medical research ought to take requires three elements discussed above:

1) The criterion, which for us will be the expectation of life at age zero.

2) The effect on this criterion of a 1 percent diminution of mortality from any cause, say $H^{(cancer)}$.

3) The effect, say $\delta^{(cancer)}$, of a given expenditure in reducing mortality from the given cause.

Having these elements for two causes, say cancer and heart disease, to each of which is associated the quantities H and δ, we can say that, if the products stand in the relation

$$H^{(cancer)}\delta^{(cancer)} > H^{(heart)}\delta^{(heart)} \ ,$$

then research ought to be devoted to cancer; if the inequality goes the other way, to heart disease.

We have thus found a guide to the strategy of medical research. Indeed, the above inequality can go beyond medicine; it can tell whether more fire stations ought to be built; whether airbags in cars ought to be mandatory; or whether prehospital attention ought to be provided for coronary patients.

But the solution remains merely formal until we know the qualities H and δ. We have seen the difficulties in regard to H, arising, despite an abundance of statistics, from our ignorance of the degree of heterogeneity in the population at a given age and sex. We can only assert that, for most causes, H is smaller than here stated, because of this heterogeneity within age-sex groups.

It is even more difficult to set a number for the result δ of a given expenditure. Millions of dollars can be spent on research without obtaining any new scientific knowledge. And even if scientific knowledge is obtained, it may not be of a kind that has direct application to saving life. The question of how much research is needed to gain the knowledge that will reduce the deaths from a given cause by 1 percent is not easy, but some suggestions may be obtained from study of medical history.

A further issue relates to classification. The causes of death here recognized are traditional medical entities in their up-to-date definitions, as incorporated in the International List of Causes of Death. They are in line with medical diagnostic practice, and are appropriate classes for treatment on present knowledge. But the quantity H is becoming smaller and smaller. In 1930 it was over 0.30 for United States males; for Swedish females today it is about 0.10. The trend suggests that it will decline further. The progress of medicine is moving us towards the point where everyone dies at about the same age, say 75 or 80.

This means a diminishing return on curative effort. More expensive equipment added to the arsenal gives smaller incremental effects. One possible explanation of these diminishing returns is that the entities being attacked are no longer the appropriate ones. It could be that cancer of the various organs, coronary attacks, stroke, and other cardiovascular causes are all manifestations of one single ailment, a general deterioration with age of the cells of the human body. No one would have made such a suggestion a century ago, when bacterial and viral diseases were the immediate preoccupation. Learning to cure these had a large effect on expectation of life, since many years separated them from the diseases of old age. We now seem to be in a new phase, with similar incidence of the several diseases by age, sex, and other characteristics. This paper has attempted to define the new phase of mortality analysis. The non-medical considerations here presented can hardly provide definitive policies for medical research. My object is to help clarify certain issues, and to learn what sorts of data would enable better decisions to be made.

Acknowledgments

I am grateful for discussion and correspondence to Joel
E. Cohen, Lloyd Demetrius, George Hutchison, George C. Myers,
Donald Shepard, and Richard Zeckhauser, each of whom has
carried one part or another of the theme of this paper
farther than I have.

References

Bernstein, Jeremy. "Profiles: Biology Watcher." The New
Yorker (January 2, 1978): 27-46.

Cohen, Joel E. "Livelihood Benefits of Small Improvements
in the Life Table." Health Services Research (Spring,
1975): 82-96.

Demetrius, Lloyd. "Relations Between Demographic Para-
meters." Unpublished manuscript, 1977.

Dubos, Rene. Mirage of Health: Utopias, Progress, and
Biological Change. New York: Harper & Row, 1959.

Keyfitz, Nathan. "What Difference Would It Make If Cancer
Were Eradicated? An Examination of the Taeuber
Paradox." Demography 14 (1977): 411-418.

McKeown, Thomas. The Modern Rise of Population. London:
Edward Arnold, 1976.

Pitts, Alfred M. Some Notes on the Collection of U.S.
Multiple Cause of Death Data with Illustrative Multiple
Cause Tabulations for 1969. Durham, North Carolina:
Duke University Center for Demographic Studies.

Preston, Samuel H., Nathan Keyfitz, and Robert Schoen.
Causes of Death: Life Tables for National Populations.
New York: Seminar Press, 1972.

Shepard, Donald S. Prediction and Incentives in Health Care
Policy. Doctoral dissertation, John Fitzgerald Kennedy
School of Government. Cambridge, Massachusetts:
Harvard University, 1976.

2. Industrialization and Economic Growth: Estimates of Their Effects on the Health of Populations

Overview

A question of primary practical and scientific importance at the present time concerns the role of economic
development in health. This question bears not only on the
conditions of populations in developing economies, but
increasingly on those in the highly industrialized countries
as well. The major concerns of the less developed nations
revolve around nutrition, housing, rapidly expanding populations, especially in urban areas, and highly skewed income
distributions (World Bank, 1978). The industrialized countries, on the other hand, appear more concerned with economic
instability--especially unemployment and very rapid economic
growth in specific regions--and industrial pollution
(Lilienfeld and Gifford, 1966; Lave and Seskin, 1977).

The research literature closely reflects these concerns.
From the international perspective, cross-sectional studies
have shown strongly and consistently inverse relations
between national levels of income and infant mortality, mortality at 1-4 years of age, and total mortality (Adelman,
1963). Recently, data have been assembled to show that the
strong inverse relation between national wealth and mortality
has been declining within the last forty years (Preston,
1976). Indeed these data appear to indicate that this traditional relationship now applies largely to non-industrial-
ized nations.

It is clear from a very long tradition of cross-sectional research in industrialized countries, however, that
the primary relationship of economic position to health
remains important up to the present time. Indeed, probably
the most consistent findings in the epidemiology of health
problems and mortality rates are their generally inverse
relation to socioeconomic status (Appendices I, II).

It has been suggested that the reason for the relative decline in the importance of national income to the health of industrialized countries involves both a sharp diminution of the beneficial impact of economic growth as well as the actual contribution of economic growth to specific health problems. Thus, in the industrialized countries, where infectious diseases are no longer an important source of mortality, the value for health of added nutrition is in question. Similarly, it is plausible that after the population's average age reaches a critical level, given a relatively fixed life span for the human species, any increases in life expectancy would occur only at dramatically higher levels of technological sophistication--if at all (Keyfitz, 1978).

Frederiksen has shown the relatively simple and clear inverse relations between changes in average national income and those in mortality for developing countries (Frederiksen, 1969). By contrast, Brenner shows that this relationship becomes highly complex in industrialized societies and, while strong, must be measured with statistical controls for multiple factors which also influence mortality patterns (Brenner, 1976; Brenner, 1979). Indeed, it appears that we are beginning to approach the point where, in industrialized countries, the problems of economic instability (unemployment and very sharp economic growth) are equal to the benefits of economic growth.

Why should economic instability act as such an important counterweight to the beneficial effects of long-term economic growth? The answers are probably to be found in those research literatures which deal with the stress of economic and social change. The literature on diffusion of innovations indicates that the dispersion of technological developments contributes to economic growth under conditions of conflict (Rogers, 1962; Smelser, 1963). These conflicts represent resistance to adoption of new procedures. The conflicts can also be seen in the literature on organizational growth (Johns, 1973; Starbuck, 1965) and on small group processes (Bales, 1966; Slater, 1966; Mills, 1964).

During periods of rapid economic growth--periods of substantial capital investment and accelerated diffusion of technological processes--many people enter new, and as yet risky, employment situations. These are moderately stressful periods--especially the "crisis" period of the economic cycle heralding a slowdown in economic growth--which also tend to involve change of residence and are associated with new family formation. Recessional periods, on the other hand, involve both short- and long-term stresses, involving both losses of income and employment, and include emotional pressures on the family and political systems. Substantial research literatures have been devoted to the stressful effects of changes in the social structure on health. In the sociological tradition these effects are identified with the theories of anomie advanced by Durkheim (1897), while in the psychological-psychiatric traditions they are associated with the original theses of Meyer (1951), Alexander (1950), and Selye (1956).

In this paper a model is presented which attempts to delineate the beneficial as well as the detrimental aspects of economic growth as they tend to influence health. The long-term, and apparently beneficial, aspects of economic growth include growth in real per capita income and income distribution via welfare transfer payments, and educational level. The stressful effects of economic change, which are associated primarily with economic instability, include rapid economic growth (measured by the residual variation in real per capita income when the smooth long-term trend is excluded) and unemployment. It is further assumed that inflation, to the extent that it affects health, does so largely by inflicting damage on the economic growth rate or by acting to maintain or increase the unemployment rate.

This model is tested on United States data for mortality rates since 1909 classified by age. The overall validity of the model is sustained by the empirical tests based on multiple regression analysis. This model is useful in specifying the main factors underlying the apparent decline in the beneficial effects of economic growth for health in industrialized societies.

Background

This paper is concerned specifically with the impact of industrialization and economic growth on the health of people in industrialized societies. We are focusing on these countries because (1) they possess the most reliable data concerning mortality; and (2) it is in these countries that one finds the largest body of studies on the relation of socioeconomic position to health status. These studies have had an extensive history and continue up to the present, especially in the United States and the United Kingdom.

The research in this area can be traced back to the 1930's in the United States. Until very recently, the majority of this research was concerned with the inverse relationship between socioeconomic status and mental and physical disorders. In other words, the research on this subject has shown higher rates of morbidity and mortality due to physical disorders, and a shorter life expectancy, among lower socioeconomic groups (Appendix I). For the mental disorders, and for indices of poor mental health, there is a similarly consistent inverse relationship between prevalence rates and socioeconomic status (Appendix II). For both physical and mental disorders, in general, there is a considerably lower rate of utilization of health care services by lower socioeconomic groups, controlling for age and levels of severity of illness, although this appears to be changing rapidly (Appendix III).

These conclusions have led to the question of the probable dynamics of the inverse relationship between socioeconomic status and health status. The generally accepted hypothesis among specialists in this field is that three factors are largely responsible for this inverse relationship:

(1) comparatively low levels of nutrition among low socioeconomic status groups, which are especially significant in the acute and chronic infectious diseases;

(2) higher levels of social-psychological stress in lower socioeconomic groups, which are particularly relevant to mental disorders, alcoholism, psychosomatic disorders, cardiovascular-renal diseases involving hypertension, and suicide, homicide, and accidents; and

(3) lower utilization of health services among lower socioeconomic groups, which is especially important in maternal and child illnesses, accidents, and cancer and malignant tumors, especially those of the female reproductive system.

With these three general factors as background, a series of studies was developed over the last fifteen years to determine the effects of adverse changes in the national economy on health status. Given the consistent findings of the substantial literature on the subject, there is reason to believe that declines in employment and income, and increased inflation, would decrease the actual socioeconomic status of significant minorities of the general population. These decreases in socioeconomic status, in turn, would lead to lowered nutrition levels, a substantially greater prevalence of social-psychological stress and decreased financial ability to utilize medical care facilities. These three factors, originating in national economic instabilities, would then have a substantial negative impact on the health of the population.

The empirical evidence strongly supports these hypotheses for both industrialized and developing countries. For
developing countries where the major sources of mortality are
the infectious diseases, and in industrialized countries for
both infectious diseases and infant and maternal illnesses,
strong inverse relationships have been observed between
national economic indicators and mortality rates (Appendix
IV, Nos. 5, 10, 11). Mortality due to the chronic diseases
has also been found to have a strong inverse relationship to
national economic indicators in industrialized countries
(Appendix IV; Brenner, 1976). These chronic diseases
include heart, cerebrovascular, and renal diseases which com-
prise the great majority of sources of mortality in these
countries. Finally, hospitalization for mental disorders has
been shown to be strongly inversely related to adverse
national economic fluctuations, as have mortality due to
alcoholism (cirrhosis of the liver), automobile accidents,
and suicide and homicide (Appendix IV, Nos. 4, 7, 8, 13).
Thus, a strong inverse relationship between changes in economic conditions and health status is apparent for a number
of countries, periods, and alternative measures of health
status.

The persistence of these findings up to the most recent
years for which data are available is especially remarkable,
if not paradoxical, when one considers a wide variety of
empirical trend data which seem to suggest that economic factors may have ceased to influence mortality significantly.
These trends, as observed in the industrialized countries,
include: (1) the near disappearance of infectious diseases--
those which are allegedly most heavily influenced by the
economy, especially through nutrition--as important causes of
mortality; (2) a sharp curtailment in the slope of decline
in mortality rates since 1950, despite higher average rates
of economic growth than occurred in the previous two decades;
(3) recent international comparative studies showing the
effect of GNP on mortality rates to have declined precipitously between 1930 and 1960 (Preston, 1976); (4) central
government efforts, especially since the great depression
and World War II, to supplement the income of lower income
groups through welfare payments, social security benefits,
and unemployment insurance (Anderson, O.W., 1972);
(5) recent evidence that the gaps in access to health care
between the lowest and highest income groups have considerably lessened, especially considering central government supported health insurance plans (U.S. Social Security Administration, 1978); (6) increasing evidence that industrial
pollution of air and water, chemical industrial occupational
hazards, and pesticides, and food additives are risk factors
in chronic disease mortality; and (7) evidence that

elements of the "affluent lifestyle" including obesity, lack
of exercise, and the use of alcohol, tobacco, and even auto-
mobiles constitute mortality risks (Lilienfeld and Gifford,
1966).

Indeed, given the significant implication for health of
these trends, one might be drawn to the conclusion that
industrialization and a comparatively high level of national
income signal the end of the traditional inverse relation
between socioeconomic status and health status. How, then,
is the apparent paradox of continuance of this inverse relation in the face of comparative national affluence to be
resolved? The answer suggested in this paper is that the
basic inverse relation between socioeconomic status and
health status can only be understood dynamically; a fundamental problem of living among lower socioeconomic groups
lies in their continuously high exposure to the instabilities
of national economic change.

Economic instabilities are characterized by a particular
relation to the ordinary processes of economic growth which
are typical of the affluent industrialized countries based on
market economies. In these countries the pattern of economic
growth is inherently unstable in that it incorporates "business cycle" fluctuations as well as longer-term sociopolitical changes. These instabilities engender the following
types of stress: (1) loss, or fear of loss, of employment or
income associated with economic recession and liquidation or
with obsolescence of technology and human skills; (2) relative deprivation of income or social status gains by specified minorities, in comparison with the majority of the
society, during periods of both rapid economic growth (i.e.,
the "prosperity" stage of the business cycle) and long-term
growth; and (3) extreme anxiety occurring at the peak of
the business cycle--called the "crisis"--which is the point
of highest earnings and lowest unemployment, but which is
immediately followed by a period of liquidation and then by
recession.

Individuals at the lowest socioeconomic levels of
society are at highest risk of exposure to these short- and
long-term economic disturbances. The reason for their unusual vulnerability lies, first of all, in their comparatively
low levels of technologically sophisticated job skills. This
comparative "lack of skill" means that they are among the
first fired during recessions and last hired during periods
of recovery. Workers of comparatively low technological
skill are also obviously the lowest paid and most heavily
unemployed in the highly sophisticated post-industrial
society. In addition, being the poorest paid and most

frequently unemployed groups in the society, the lower socioeconomic groups possess the fewest resources with which to
combat the actuality or fear of loss, or the frustration of
deprivation relative to the rest of the society.

There are several traditions of theory and research
which deal with the social stress involved in economic
changes. The largest research literature on this subject is
found in sociology. Indeed, this subject has been one of the
core interests of sociological thinkers.

The original delineation of the stressful effects of
economic fluctuations in the sociological tradition is attributed to Durkheim in his classic study of suicide (1897).
Durkheim argued that suicide is one of the most acute and
dramatic reactions of individuals to a state of "anomie".
Anomie, in turn, is a condition resulting from a comparative
absence of integration of the social structure, and leads to
a breakdown in normative patterns of behavior. Among the
most important phenomena which precipitate declines in social
integration are changes in the economic situation, regardless
of whether depressed or prosperous conditions occur.

Perhaps the best known interpretation of the Durkheimian
conception of anomie is that of Merton (1957). Merton's formulation translates anomie through the concepts of culture
and social structure--concepts which are among the basic components of modern sociological theory. Thus, for Merton anomie represents a condition of disjuncture of cultural demands
and social structural realities. The typical anomic situation, then, occurs when an individual's economic position,
which depends on the behavior of the aggregate economic system, is at variance with a dignified lifestyle as defined by
the values and norms of the culture. Kleiner and Parker
(1963) have further defined this situation, on the individual level, as the difference between aspirations and achievement.

Other sociological writers have identified additional
sources of poor social integration (Parsons, 1951; Dodge and
Martin, 1970; Moss, 1973), including some which are observa-
ble at the individual level (Lenski, 1954; Gross, 1970). Of
these, Lenski's formulation of "status integration" has perhaps been one of the most productive of sociological research
on stress (e.g., Jackson, 1962). In Lenski's conception,
poor status integration, and therefore stress, occurs when
any of the characteristics of a person's social position
(e.g., educational level, occupation, income, ethnicity) is
not closely interconnected with one or more of the other
parts. In a typical example, an individual has attained

income or employment above or below the level that his educational or ethnic background would have normally predicted.
From a time-oriented, or dynamic, perspective, the common
denominator that emerges as the source of poor social inte-
gration--which, in turn, results in stress--is social mobility. In the delineation of social mobility, we are including not only downward and upward movements in social position but also "relative mobility" and fear of downward mobility. Relative downward mobility, for example, refers to
situations where the subject loses status as a result of the
fact that others of his age or socioeconomic status have
moved upward while he has failed to do so. Fear of downward
mobility frequently occurs where the subject has actually
experienced upward mobility, e.g., a promotion, but the challenge and risk inherent in the new, higher status position
bring about anxiety over the possibility of failure.

For many students of the behavior of humans and other
social animals, it may be intuitive that the basic source of
societal stress is a lack of social integration (Cassel,
1970; Caplan, et. al., 1977). Those for whom this idea is
intuitive will require no further explanation of the relation
of poor social integration to a variety of pathologies. In
that intuitive sociological sense, "attachment", "relationship", or "belongingness" is the basis of life for all social
animals. Some indeed may refer to these expressions of
social integration as fundamental "needs". Others, however,
may require an explanation which links the sociological to
the psychological perspective. Such an explanation is provided, for example, by Blau who has developed a theoretical
framework for viewing social relationships as exchange networks (Blau, 1964). In this perspective, it is through
social relations that all things of value are exchanged, from
the most basic goods and services to abstract conceptions and
emotion-laden symbols. Moving even closer to the psychological domain, it is possible with a behaviorally-oriented
sociological perspective (Burgess and Bushell, 1969) such as
that of Homans (1961) to envisage social exchange systems as
the basic structure of society which exercise social control
under principles of learning theory.

Moreover, when we move from the macrosocietal to the
individual level of analysis, we find a remarkably consistent
view of stress which is based on the frequency of life
changes. The germinal formulation of Selye in 1956 suggested
that the phenomenon of change itself--beyond the capacities
of the organism to adapt--is the critical precipitant of
pathology (Selye, 1956). This formulation has been the guiding concept for a large number of researchers into the stress-
producing potential of different types of life changes. For

example, in summarizing the theoretical orientation of many
researchers in this field, Levi indicates that the highest
stress levels are usually found at the extremes of the stimu-
lation continuum and thus deprivation or excess of almost any
influence is provocative of stress (Levi, 1972).

However, the research evidence from studies on mental
disorder (Mueller, et al., 1977), especially depression
(Paykel, 1974), and criminal behavior (Gersten, et al., 1974)
indicates clearly that life changes viewed as undesirable
show considerably greater potency to provoke pathological
responses. When one includes traditional research pioneered
by Holmes and Rahe using weighted life change scales (Holmes
and Rahe, 1967) and showing chronic disease reactions within
a 2-year lag period of cumulative stresses (Holmes and
Masuda, 1974), the weight of the evidence, is that, while all
significant life changes are potential stressors, undesirable
changes are predictive of higher stress levels. If this perspective is correct, then we should observe that economic
recession shows more severe and longer lasting pathological
effects than periods of rapid economic growth; but the
periods of growth themselves, while desirable for their long-
term implications, nevertheless are stressful.

A related issue, which the stress literature does not
deal with systematically, is that of the inter-relation among
life changes. The guiding hypothesis of the formulation in
the present study is that deleterious life changes in particular are capable of producing stresses which in turn lead to
other life changes and stresses. This interaction among
stresses has been labelled the principle of acceleration of
stress (Brenner, 1979). An example would be the loss of a
job, which may lead to financial disruption, marital and
parent-child strains and possibly the breakup of family,
possible loss of friendships which were employment-related,
the securing of a new job and at a lower status, with the
requirement of moving to a residence in a new area in order
to manage the job. In this formulation, the more undesirable
the life change, the greater the probability of additional
life changes or stressors. It is clear from the principle
of acceleration of stress, that job and income loss are
particularly productive of stressful changes. Are there
aspects of rapid economic growth, however, which while not
usually accelerative in their stressful impact, do result in
at least discrete, short-term stresses?

Based on theories of Durkheim and Merton, Henry and
Short developed an explanation of why homicide appeared to
show a stronger association with economic upturns than with
downturns. They reasoned that since homicide was probably

primarily an expression of aggression manifested by lower socioeconomic groups, at least one primary source of stress for those groups must be associated with expanding, rather than contracting, economic activity. Henry and Short concluded that this source of stress for lower socioeconomic groups was the relative deprivation brought about in periods in which the majority of the population significantly improved their economic situations while the lowest socioeconomic groups, who gained in absolute terms, suffered in relative terms (Henry and Short, 1954).

The argument presented in this paper takes the Henry and Short position a step further. Those socioeconomic groups most likely to experience relative deprivation during the economic upturns have probably also been thrust into a somewhat lower socioeconomic postion as a result of the previous recession. This would be true, in any case, because lower socioeconomic groups have the highest unemployment rates during recessional periods.

A related point is based on the fact that the economic "upturn" or "expansion" is simply the period of most rapid acceleration of general, or long-term, economic growth. More broadly speaking, it is the period of most acute and sweeping social change within the longer-term social trends dependent on technological developments. It is within these cyclic upturns in the economy that the greatest investment in, and manifestation of, technological innovation (including its accompanying social structural developments) occurs. This period of rapid cultural change, in economies which show the typical long-term growth pattern, is especially difficult on the (a) unskilled, (b) older workers, (c) the aged, and (d) other individuals who have the deepest investment in the status quo.

Finally, both low and high socioeconomic status groups experience the stress phenomenon occurring at the "peak" or "crisis" point in the economic cycle and resulting from a radical departure of the economic situation from expecta-tions (not only aspirations) of continuing rapid growth. This is also a situation of relatively high income (prosperity) at a time when for a significant number of persons the economic situation is worsening--thus engendering absolute and relative deprivation for a significant proportion of both high and low socioeconomic status groups.

If, as we suggest, the short-term stresses of rapid economic growth are discrete rather than cumulative, how might they influence mortality within a short period? Clearly, they could do so only if they occurred close to the end of a period of successive stresses in which the principle of acceleration was operating. This means, in effect, that only persons predisposed through the earlier experience of a cumulative series of stresses, would be at risk of stress-induced mortality associated with the short term stresses of rapid economic growth.

The individuals, therefore, at highest risk of mortality associated with rapid economic growth probably have within the previous two years experienced a cumulative series of stresses (Brenner, 1979). The individuals most likely to have had such experiences are those who lost employment or substantial income during the previous recession. We may conclude, then, that the significant downgrading of social position not only (1) engenders a series of stresses through an acceleration process and (2) depletes resources that could otherwise be used to cope with stresses, but, (3) makes the individual unusually susceptible to new stresses which arise subsequently, but are frequently related to the original downgrading of social position.

Thus, by virtue of the experience of loss stemming from recession, individuals are more likely to suffer the additional stresses of relative deprivation associated with "prosperity", and shocked frustration inherent in the "crisis" period. We then have a set of situations of sequential, and additive stresses--namely, severe loss--relative deprivation--shock and frustration--which, in sum, make for the greatest overall risk to health. A relatively common example of this sequence might involve a person forty years of age who lost employment after having accumulated seniority. His next job might well be at a place where he has no seniority, is supervised by younger and less experienced workers and--especially because of his age and newness to the job--must work particularly hard to demonstrate his capabilities. His experience of the relative deprivation of a comparatively low status in relation to his earlier position and to those of his new peers and superordinates will be seriously compounded if his hopes for a more stable future are dashed by the "crisis" which spells an end to the growth of the firm in which he now works.

Methods

We examine the relationship between national economic changes and age-specific mortality rates for the United States over the period 1909-1976, excluding 1918--the year of the international influenza pandemic. The year 1909 is selected as the first year for the study because only by then were at least twenty states included in the United

States mortality statistics. Four central independent variables are utilized to explain trend variations in the age-
specific mortality rates: (1) the long-term trend in
economic growth; (2) government expenditures for welfare
payments; (3) the unemployment rate; and (4) comparatively
rapid economic growth.

The long-term trend in economic growth is measured by
estimating the exponential trend in per-capita personal
income in constant dollars--i.e., controlling for the effects
of inflation. Welfare payments by government are computed
as a proportion of total government expenditures (Appendix
V, No. 1). We do not use the absolute amount spent by
government on welfare as the indicator because welfare
expenditures, especially over the long trend, are highly
correlated with total government expenditures. Thus, the
variable absolute-welfare-payment might tend to reflect the
overall magnitude of industrial activity that is based on,
or influenced by, governmental effort. We control for this
potential influence on our data by dividing government welfare expenditures by total government expenditures.

Prior to 1940, our unemployment figures represent estimates of unemployment on as comparable a basis to current
labor force concepts as is presently possible. There have
been many estimates of unemployment for these years prepared
by such agencies as the National Industrial Conference Board.
In all of these, included the series used here, unemployment
is calculated as a residual. That is, estimates are first
made of the civilian labor force, then of employment; the
difference between the two provides the estimates of unemployment. The figures for decennial census years are used
as benchmarks, with interpolations made for intercensal years
from a variety of available sources (Appendix V, No. 3;
Source 1, Part 1, p. 124).

Comparatively rapid economic growth describes the
"cyclic" phasing of the economic growth process. The
cyclic phases of economic growth involve a recurring
succession of business activities, loosely divisible into
periods of prosperity, crisis, liquidation, recession, and
recovery (Webster, 1971, p. 362). The higher values of the
rapid economic growth variable are observed during the prosperity phase, with the very highest values occurring at the
crisis phase. The crisis phase is, therefore, the culminating point of business prosperity, with the lowest rates
of unemployment, after which economic growth slows considerably, and a period of liquidation ensues (Webster, 1971,
Crisis No. 5, p. 629). As economic growth continues to slow,
the period of recession with the highest rates of unemployment and greatest losses of income, sets in. The period of

recession thus includes the lowest values of economic growth. The recovery period begins as economic growth once again begins to quicken and subsequently to go into its comparatively rapid phase.

In order to measure this cyclic component of economic growth, we use the traditional method of detrending the overall measure of economic growth. Thus, comparatively rapid economic growth is estimated by the residual variation--i.e., the fluctuation remaining--in real per-capita income after it has been detrended of the exponential long-term growth trend described above. We refer to this variable as indicating comparatively rapid economic growth, namely the crisis periods. Its lowest, and therefore, negative, values represent the periods of slowest economic growth which also correspond to (but are not perfectly inversely correlated with) the period's highest unemployment rates.

The long-term exponential trend of economic growth should show an inverse relation to mortality, since it is this growth in real wealth which over the long run makes it possible for the society to provide basic economic security and to invest in medical research, and health manpower and facilities. The magnitude of welfare payments, in proportion to other government expenditures, reflects over the long term the extent of dependency of the citizenry on government for their living expenses and health care.

Over the long term, the proportion of elderly and chronically ill in need of basic support and health care has tended to increase with the average age of the population. To the extent that welfare expenditures indicate the degree of support required by the population, the relation to mortality rates should be positive since the welfare variable is describing situations of very low income and perhaps unemployment.

The study hypotheses argue for separating two main groups of cyclic phases of economic growth in terms of their stressful effects. The impact of the liquidation and recession periods is indicated by the unemployment rate which increases during the liquidation period and reaches its peak during the recessional period. We expect that the impact of this highly stressful period occurs over a period of several years. This group of stresses, involving fundamental losses of social position, income, and other resources, sets off in an accelerated fashion a series of additional stresses. The stress research literature based on life change analysis indicates an average duration of

two years between the first of a series of cumulative
stresses and the onset of serious illness (Rahe et al.,
1964). We expect, then, that increased mortality rates
should lag behind increased unemployment rates by at least
an average of two years. The entire lag of the increased
mortality behind increased unemployment might range for a
considerably longer time span. We have difficulty in measuring that lagged effect of mortality behind unemployment
beyond five years because the entire duration of economic
growth cycles is hardly ever more than five years. Therefore, it is argued that the relationship between unemployment and mortality rates should be observed within the
2-to-5 year period following the increased unemployment
rates, while the average or "peak" effect should be observed
at approximately the two-year lag.

The recovery-prosperity and crisis phases, indicating
the short-term discrete stresses, respectively, of relative
deprivation and acute anxiety, are represented in the positive values of the rapid economic growth variable. We
expect, therefore, that these short-term discrete stresses
will influence mortality only in the population that is
highly predisposed to mortality as a result of a long
series of previously experienced stresses--typically
originating in the earlier recessional period of economic
loss. Thus, the increased mortality associated with rapid
economic growth may be seen within a year of the incidence
of the discrete stress involved.

We shall test the overall hypotheses simultaneously by
including variables representing each hypothesis in a single
multiple regression model for time-series analysis. There
is a problem in using the time-series approach to regression
analysis of economic and mortality data, because of the
potential--extremely common in time-series approaches--of
correlated regression residuals which can greatly bias the
resulting coefficients and tests of statistical significance.

One of the main reasons for the existence of correlated
residuals in time-series regressions is the fact that each
time-series is itself often serially correlated--i.e., each
observation is somewhat predictable from the preceding one
and thus the observations do not reflect the true independence that is required for the testing of statistical
significance. This problem of lack of independence of
observations is typical of both economic and mortality data.
Both types of data evidence trends and cycles--or smooth
movements through which each observation is partly predicted
by the earlier observation or set of observations.

Fortunately, over the past two decades, tests for the presence of correlated residuals and methods of data transformation to remedy this problem have become widely used. In this study we use the Durbin-Watson statistic (Durbin and Watson, 1950) to measure correlated residuals, and the Cochrane-Orcutt transformation (Cochrane and Orcutt, 1949) to minimize bias. One of the more important features of this data transformation, which several other popular types also possess, involves the conversion of the data to their first differences--or, in our case, to annual changes. This procedure is one of the best known and simplest techniques for minimizing trends or cyclic movements without destroying the basic validity and internal structure of the original data.

Since recessional economic activity--as measured by the unemployment rate--is hypothesized to influence general mortality rates starting on average at a two-year lag following increased unemployment, and lasting at least four years, the standard polynomial distributed lag technique can be used (Schmidt and Wand, 1973). We thus estimate the relation between mortality rates and unemployment rates, when the consequences of the latter are estimated over the period of two to five years' lag.

An additional set of tests are run in order to estimate the individual year showing the most highly predictable lag of mortality behind unemployment, examining the lags of one to five years. The chronologically synchronous relation of unemployment to mortality at lag = 0 is not estimated, because unemployment at lag zero is occasionally inversely correlated with the rapid economic growth variable at lag zero. We therefore infer that the association between unemployment and mortality is often the inverse of the association between rapid economic growth and mortality. Thus, insofar as unemployment at lag zero is incorporated statistically in our equation by virtue of its occasional inverse relation to the rapid economic growth variable, we have already obtained its estimated association with the mortality rate.

Finally, after finding the single year which provides the best lag prediction for the relation between unemployment and mortality, we restate the equations using unemployment at the optimal year among the individual one to five years of lag. This is done in order to obtain the most simple, and easily reproducible prediction equation for the mortality rates.

Table 1

MULTIPLE REGRESSION EQUATIONS OF NATIONAL ECONOMIC INDICES ON AGE-SPECIFIC MORTALITY RATES, UNITED STATES, 1909-76.[1] Regression Estimates for Unemployment Rate Based on Sum of Lagged Coefficients Over 2-5 Years, Calculated With Polynomial Distributed Lag Function[Δ]

Mortality Age Groups	Intercept	% Govt Expend on Welfare From Total Expend	Exponent Trend Long Term Long Term Per Capita Income	Residuals From Long Term Per Capita Income[2]	Unemployment Rate, Lags 2-5 Years	Coefficic of Determination R^2	Durbin-Watson Statistic	Statistical significance of Equation F	1st Order Serial Coeff Rho
Total	11.207 (8.491)**	0.021 (2.628)**	-0.001 (-1.911)*	0.002 (5.00)**	4.502 (1.892)*	0.9812	2.465	425.581	0.928 (20.059)**
Infant	70.990 (4.754)**	0.101 (1.122)	-0.015 (-3.191)**	0.012 (3.014)**	41.044 (1.531)+	0.992	2.455	996.164	0.926 (19.815)**
Ages 1-4	3.835 (1.505)+	0.012 (0.787)	-0.001 (-1.238)	0.002 (2.981)**	6.137 (1.34)+	0.984	2.521	491.737	0.927 (19.984)**
Ages 5-9	1.265 (2.110)*	0.001 (0.409)	-0.0003 (-1.523)+	0.0002 (1.659)+	1.261 (1.337)+	0.989	2.145	741.597	0.938 (21.748)**

** .01 Level of Significance
* .05 Level of Significance
+ .10 Level of Significance
[1] 1918, the year of the international influenza pandemic, was removed from the analysis.
[2] Indicator of rapid economic growth.
[Δ] Regressions based on Cochran-Orcutt data transformations.

Table 1. (continued)

Age Groups	Intercept	Welfare Expend	Exponent Trend	Residuals	Unemployment	R^2	D.W.	F	Rho
Ages 10-14	1.297 (3.626)**	0.002 (0.730)	-0.0003 (-2.481)**	0.0002 (2.238)*	0.826 (1.335)+	0.991	2.090	851.184	0.931 (20.628)**
Ages 15-19	1.992 (3.113)**	0.002 (0.452)	-0.0003 (-1.607)+	0.001 (3.876)**	1.913 (1.605)+	0.986	1.890	571.068	0.925 (19.642)**
Ages 20-24	2.441 (2.317)**	0.005 (0.804)	-0.0004 (-1.062)	0.001 (3.740)**	2.357 (1.306)	0.985	1.695	516.083	0.933 (20.916)**
Ages 25-29	2.612 (2.368)*	0.008 (1.123)	-0.0004 (-1.232)	0.001 (3.338)**	3.604 (1.711)*	0.984	1.558	510.021	0.923 (19.354)**
Ages 30-34	3.153 (2.367)*	0.008 (0.989)	-0.001 (-1.138)	0.001 (3.795)**	3.335 (1.394)+	0.984	1.770	492.859	0.928 (20.034)**
Ages 35-39	4.271 (2.952)**	0.010 (1.280)	-0.653 (-1.455)+	0.001 (3.729)**	3.315 (1.462)+	0.988	1.960	680.291	0.938 (21.895)**
Ages 40-44	7.133 (3.694)**	0.010 (1.438)+	-0.001 (-2.193)*	0.001 (3.574)**	4.123 (1.835)*	0.990	2.074	810.208	0.955 (25.844)**
Ages 45-49	11.599 (9.051)**	0.011 (1.278)	-0.002 (-4.458)**	0.001 (2.949)**	4.084 (1.574)+	0.988	2.223	653.828	0.918 (18.669)**

** .01 Level of Significance

* .05 Level of Significance

+ .10 Level of Significance

Table 1. (continued)

Age Groups	Intercept	Welfare Expend	Exponent Trend	Residuals	Unemployment	R^2	D.W.	F	Rho
Ages 50-54	16.906 (9.888)**	0.016 (1.505)+	-0.002 (-4.472)	0.002 (3.366)**	4.658 (1.434)+	0.985	2.231	522.982	0.921 (19.07)**
Ages 55-59	24.897 (9.834)**	0.020 (1.466)+	-0.003 (-4.382)**	0.003 (4.306)**	4.606 (1.091)	0.985	2.350	517.321	0.931 (20.493)**
Ages 60-64	34.393 (23.425)**	0.035 (1.757)*	-0.004 (-8.477)**	0.003 (3.094)**	3.542 (0.665)	0.981	2.524	412.318	0.829 (11.938)**
Ages 65-69	47.204 (10.188)**	0.053 (1.601)+	-0.005 (-3.543)**	0.005 (3.585)**	0.143 (0.009)	0.9805	2.535	409.77	0.915 (18.236)**
Ages 70-74	79.006 (10.514)**	0.096 (1.796)*	-0.011 (-4.249)**	0.007 (3.129)**	0.143 (0.009)	0.981	2.535	409.768	0.911 (17.864)**
Ages 75-79	122.468 (20.242)**	0.322 (3.335)**	-0.020 (-9.119)**	0.007 (1.662)+	121.918 (4.928)**	0.979	2.038	373.185	0.795 (10.584)**
Ages 80-84	190.714 (17.833)**	0.443 (2.402)**	-0.031 (-7.887)**	0.014 (1.816)*	193.508 (4.208)**	0.966	1.821	233.019	0.775 (9.883)**
Ages 85+	285.248 (21.466)**	0.934 (3.214)**	-0.042 (-8.338)**	0.038 (3.373)**	253.515 (3.896)**	0.952	1.917	160.496	0.704 (8.002)**

** .01 Level of Significance   + .10 Level of Significance
* .05 Level of Significance

Findings

Equations used in the multivariate regression analyses over the period 1909-76 are presented in Tables 1, 2 and 3. / The general pattern of findings shown in all of these tables is similar. The two cyclic influences of economic change, namely, rapid economic growth and recession (as measured by the unemployment rate) coexist. That is, they show statistically significant and independent, additive relations to the mortality rate in the same prediction equation. Neither of these independent relationships to mortality overpowers the other; rapid economic growth shows its impact within a few months and the impact of recession on total (i.e., not cause-specific) mortality lags by at least one year, and extends to at least a five-year lag.

The implication is that the recessional impact on mortality is by far the stronger of the two and probably initiates the 1-3 year process whereby mortality rates are ultimately increased. Since, as the stress-illness literature indicates, approximately two years are required for the impact of cumulative stresses to influence serious chronic disease mortality (Rahe et al., 1964) it is probable that the effects of rapid economic growth within one year are influencing the mortality rates only after a process of cumulative stresses has been set in motion as a result of the previous recession. Indeed, it is possible that rapid economic growth is influential in elevating the mortality rates of only those populations which have earlier experienced severe loss./ The additive relationship expressed in the equation may thus be interpreted to say that the greatest risk of increased mortality rates occurs in populations which have experienced both (1) initial economic loss and (2) subsequent relative deprivation and the destruction of hope signalled by the "crisis".

The equations presented in Tables 1, 2, and 3 also show that, over the long term, exponentially increasing economic growth and the proportion of government spending required for allocation to welfare payments, are positively associated with mortality rates. It should be kept in mind, then, that not only are the two cyclic effects of economic activity independently associated with mortality, but these cyclic effects are independent of the two long-term trend influences of the economy. All four variables independently coexist in the same equations which predict mortality rates.

Table 2

RELATIONSHIPS BETWEEN UNEMPLOYMENT RATES AND MORTALITY RATES,
BASED ON SEPARATE REGRESSION EQUATIONS IN WHICH THE EFFECT
OF UNEMPLOYMENT IS LAGGED 1-5 YEARS. Controls are Imposed
for the Variables: Government Welfare Payments, Exponential
Economic Growth Trend, and Comparatively Rapid Economic
Growth Δ

Mortality Age Groups	Unemployment 1 Yr Lag	Unemployment 2 Yr Lag	Unemployment 3 Yr Lag	Unemployment 4 Yr Lag	Unemployment 5 Yr Lag
Total	0.423 (0.256)	4.524 (3.204)**	-2.497 (-1.641)+	-0.360 (-0.236)	2.736 (1.892)*
Infant	-12.104 (-0.647)	50.926 (3.177)**	-26.198 (-1.517)+	-19.900 (-1.160)	31.674 (1.936)*
Ages 1-4	-2.189 (-0.671)	8.072 (2.850)**	-3.978 (-1.313)	-5.682 (-1.937)*	6.553 (2.328)*
Ages 5-9	-0.865 (-1.469)+	1.262 (2.392)**	0.370 (0.659)	-0.891 (-1.642)+	0.556 (1.040)
Ages 10-14	-0.240 (-0.634)	0.446 (1.293)	0.775 (2.261)*	-0.158 (-0.450)	-0.290 (-0.085)
Ages 15-19	0.196 (0.270)	0.732 (1.107)	1.130 (1.696)*	-0.066 (-0.099)	0.541 (0.834)
Ages 20-24	0.117 (0.107)	1.138 (1.145)	1.659 (1.656)+	-0.412 (-0.410)	0.483 (0.494)
Ages 25-29	0.851 (0.660)	2.021 (1.739)*	1.618 (1.352)+	-0.429 (-0.359)	1.041 (0.901)
Ages 30-34	1.387 (0.960)	1.892 (1.436)+	1.723 (1.279)	-0.696 (-0.520)	1.002 (0.771)
Ages 35-39	1.441 (1.066)	1.406 (1.133)	1.933 (1.537)+	(-0.174) (-0.138)	0.812 (0.664)
Ages 40-44	1.471 (1.095)	2.352 (1.939)*	1.382 (1.093)	-0.053 (-0.042)	1.064 (0.876)
Ages 45-49	1.974 (1.265)	2.546 (1.794)*	1.320 (0.894)	-0.204 (-0.140)	1.107 (0.783)

** .01 Level of Significance   + .10 Level of Significance
* .05 Level of Significance

Table 2. (continued)

Mortality Age Groups	Unemployment 1 Yr Lag	Unemployment 2 Yr Lag	Unemployment 3 Yr Lag	Unemployment 4 Yr Lag	Unemployment 5 Yr Lag
Ages 50-54	1.680 (0.856)	3.427 (1.942)*	1.274 (0.689)	-0.437 (-0.240)	1.061 (0.599)
Ages 55-59	4.995 (2.017)*	4.089 (1.776)*	-1.103 (-0.459)	-0.199 (-0.084)	2.041 (0.891)
Ages 60-64	7.155 (2.107)*	6.492 (2.071)*	-0.461 (-0.140)	-2.075 (-0.648)	-0.212 (-0.068)
Ages 65-69	12.077 (2.080)*	11.147 (2.081)*	-0.012 (-0.002)	0.395 (0.071)	4.769 (0.888)
Ages 70-74	21.652 (2.310)*	15.208 (1.727)*	-4.767 (-0.519)	-14.831 (-1.678)*	0.713 (0.081)
Ages 75-79	52.258 (2.849)**	46.626 (2.728)**	-3.945 (-0.216)	28.453 (1.608)+	56.725 (3.539)**
Ages 80-84	92.114 (2.734)**	92.580 (2.997)**	-1.505 (-0.045)	38.442 (1.182)	81.967 (2.716)**
Ages 85+	147.957 (2.725)**	135.227 (2.699)**	-65.110 (-1.223)	108.646 (2.189)*	153.504 (3.404)**

** .01 Level of Significance
* .05 Level of Significance
+ .10 Level of Significance
Δ Regressions based on Cochran-Orcutt data transformations.

Table 3

MULTIPLE REGRESSION EQUATIONS OF NATIONAL ECONOMIC INDICES ON AGE-SPECIFIC MORTALITY RATES, UNITED STATES, 1909-76.[1] Lag for Unemployment Rate Based on Year of Greatest Predictability for Specific Age Groups, or for the Total Population△

Mortality Age Groups	Intercept	% Govt Expend on Welfare From Total Expend	Exponent Trend Long Term Long Term Per Capita Income	Residuals From Long Term Per Capita Income	Unemployment Rate 2 Yr Lag 3 Yr Lag	Coeffic of Determination R^2	Durbin-Watson Statistic	Statistical Signif of Equation F	1st Order Serial Coeff Rho
Total	11.3735 (9.302)**	0.016 (1.996)*	-0.001 (-1.989)*	0.002 (4.680)**	4.524 (3.204)**	0.9774	2.524	647.471	0.918 (18.677)**
Infant	76.018 (5.519)**	0.030 (0.315)	-0.016 (-3.517)**	0.011 (2.662)**	50.926 (3.177)**	0.990	2.485	1497.51	0.917 (18.538)**
Ages 1-4	4.506 (1.824)*	-0.004 (-0.214)	-0.001 (-1.318)	0.002 (2.50)**	8.072 (2.850)**	0.979	2.543	687.632	0.918 (18.605)**
Ages 5-9	1.321 (2.206)*	-0.0002 (-0.513)	-0.0003 (-1.522)+	0.0002 (1.663)+	1.262 (2.392)**	0.988	2.172	1251.17	0.937 (21.638)**

** .01 Level of Significance
* .05 Level of Significance
+ .10 Level of Significance
1 1918, the year of the international influenza pandemic, was removed from the analysis.
2 Indicator of rapid economic growth.
△ Regressions based on Cochran-Orcutt data transformations.

Table 3. (continued)

Age Groups	Inter-cept	Welfare Expend	Exponent Trend	Residuals	Unemployment 2 Yr	3 Yr	R^2	D.W.	F	Rho
Ages 10-14	1.278 (3.535)**	0.001 (0.676)	-0.0003 (-2.397)**	0.0002 (2.160)*		0.775 (2.261)*	0.990	2.061	1533.88	0.934 (21.117)**
Ages 15-19	2.108 (3.383)**	0.001 (0.374)	-0.0003 (-1.711)*	0.001 (4.024)**		1.130 (1.696)*	0.986	1.927	1020.51	0.925 (19.626)**
Ages 20-24	2.283 (2.048)*	0.004 (0.718)	-0.0003 (-0.862)	0.001 (3.807)**		1.659 (1.656)+	0.984	1.747	926.487	0.937 (21.677)**
Ages 25-29	2.842 (2.626)**	0.008 (1.111)	-0.001 (-1.339)+	0.001 (3.748)**	2.021 (1.739)*		0.984	1.683	899.042	0.923 (19.284)**
Ages 30-34	3.587 (2.861)**	0.007 (0.944)	-0.001 (-1.400)+	0.001 (4.184)**	1.892 (1.436)+		0.983	1.867	869.204	0.925 (19.688)**
Ages 35-39	4.522 (3.216)**	0.009 (1.265)	-0.001 (-1.574)+	0.001 (3.862)**		1.933 (1.537)+	0.988	1.976	1220.70	0.939 (21.947)**
Ages 40-44	7.601 (4.223)**	0.011 (1.496)+	-0.001 (-2.467)**	0.001 (4.047)**	2.352 (1.939)*		0.990	2.150	1451.47	0.953 (25.321)**
Ages 45-49	11.770 (9.410)**	0.011 (1.302)	-0.002 (-4.572)**	0.001 (3.305)**	2.546 (1.794)*		0.988	2.298	1180.67	0.914 (18.552)**

** .01 Level of Significance   + .10 Level of Significance
* .05 Level of Significance

Table 3. (continued)

Age Groups	Inter-cept	Welfare Expend	Exponent Trend	Residuals	Unemployment 2 Yr	3 Yr	R^2	D.W.	F	Rho
Ages 50-54	17.083 (10.521)**	0.006 (1.518)+	-0.002 (-4.690)**	0.002 (3.689)**	3.427 (1.942)*		0.985	2.280	952.246	0.919 (18.816)**
Ages 55-59	24.846 (10.929)**	0.008 (1.334)+	-0.003 (-4.702)**	0.003 (4.504)**	4.089 (1.776)*		0.984	2.379	926.794	0.927 (19.909)**
Ages 60-64	34.133 (24.278)**	0.030 (1.632)+	-0.004 (-8.538)**	0.002 (3.055)**	6.492 (2.071)*		0.980	2.503	749.580	0.829 (11.960)**
Ages 65-69	47.595 (10.882)**	0.049 (1.566)+	-0.005 (-3.708)**	0.005 (3.847)**	11.147 (2.081)*		0.984	2.443	911.279	0.911 (17.850)**
Ages 70-74	77.746 (10.684)**	0.071 (1.370)+	-0.010 (-4.196)**	0.007 (2.887)**	15.209 (1.727)*		0.979	2.539	714.474	0.911 (17.779)**
Ages 75-79	127.716 (12.806)**	0.321 (3.194)**	-0.020 (-5.717)**	0.010 (2.243)*	46.626 (2.728)**		0.972	1.907	526.528	0.871 (14.322)**
Ages 80-84	200.13 (12.909)**	0.457 (2.503)**	-0.032 (-5.710)**	0.019 (2.339)*	92.581 (2.997)**		0.961	1.833	366.794	0.849 (12.951)**
Ages 85+	295.269 (16.640)**	0.964 (3.193)**	-0.043 (-6.433)**	0.043 (3.401)**	135.227 (2.699)**		0.939	2.029	229.599	0.775 (9.896)**

** .01 Level of Significance
* .05 Level of Significance
+ .10 Level of Significance

We can observe in Tables 1, 2, and 3, in addition, that the Durbin-Watson statistics are almost always in the appropriate range (Durbin and Watson, 1950, 1951) which indicates the absence of significant bias due to auto-correlation of regression residuals. Evidence that the Cochrane-Orcutt (1949) transformation, which minimizes regression residual autocorrelation, has been appropriately used is provided by the fact the estimate of rho (the first order serial correlation coefficient) is always statistically significant.

It is also evident that the coefficients of determination (R^2) are highly significant statistically (according to the "F" value) and are almost always above the 90 percent level. Such relatively high R^2's are not uncommon in time-series analysis in which long-term trends are part of the predictive equations. Nevertheless, the importance of these high R^2's is that a high level of predictability of mortality rates can be achieved through the use of economic indicators. Also, and perhaps more significant, is that we can be reasonably confident that no other important predictor of mortality rate trends, that is not associated with one of the variables now in the predictive equations, has been left out of the equations. This means, in turn, that the proper statistical controls necessary for estimating coefficients for each of the independent predictive variables have been operative in each of the predictive equations.

In Table 1, specifically, we find that the unemployment rate, with a distributed lag estimation of its impact over 2-5 years, shows a statistically significant relationship to mortality at the 90 per cent level of confidence for all but two age groups out of nineteen. For total mortality, as for eight of the individual age groups, the relationships are significant at the 95 per cent confidence level at least.

In Table 2, we compare the impact of the unemployment rate with a two-year lagged effect on mortality against its one-, three-, four-, and five-year lagged impacts. Our objective is to determine the extent to which the two-year lagged effect of unemployment, as would be predicted by the life-change research, is the most efficient single lag predictor for an estimate of the association between unemployment and mortality. Beyond the pragmatic issue of obtaining the single best lag estimate of the impact of unemployment on mortality, we are also interested in determining the most efficient lag predictor for theoretical reasons. Indeed, it might be argued that while unemployment should show its most potent overall effect after

Figure 1

GRAPHIC ANALYSIS OF THE RELATION BETWEEN THE
TOTAL MORTALITY RATE OF THE POPULATION AGED 55-64
AND THE EMPLOYMENT RATE,* UNITED STATES, 1909-1976

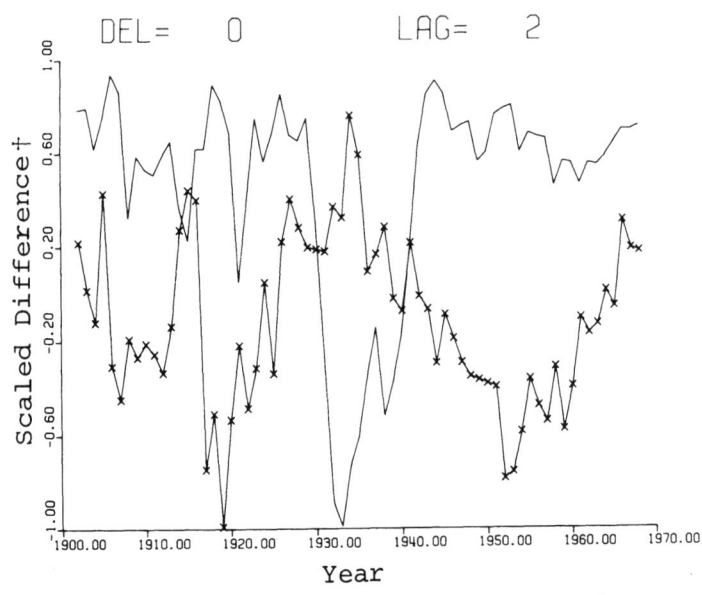

———x—x—x———   Total Mortality Rate

——————————   U.S. Unemployment Rate,
                Inverted

*Employment Rate = Inverted Unemployment Rate

†Scaled Difference: Both series are scaled for viewing such
  that the greatest amplitude from the arithmetic mean of each
  series, which is set equal to zero, has been normalized to
  +1.00 if positive, or -1.00 if negative.

Del = 0: long-term trends subtracted from the mortality
          series.
Lag = 2: mortality is lagged two years.

two years, the very oldest and youngest populations--
presumably the least resistant to potentially fatal
illnesses--would show increased mortality at considerably
less than two years after the occurrence of serious
economic loss.

Table 2 only partly bears out these hypotheses. It
appears that only the population over 55 years of age shows
the impact of unemployment on mortality after only a one
year lag. Also, it appears to be the case that the populations between ages 10 and 39, and especially between 10
and 19, show a more prominent lag of the effect of unemployment at three rather than two years. However, the
youngest age groups (under 10 years) show the peak impact
to be at two years' lag, as it is for the population as
a whole. Table 2 also shows a general lack of statistical
significance of the influence of the unemployment rate on
mortality at discrete lags after three years.

In Table 3, we show the entire prediction equations
for age-specific mortality based on the most efficient lag
for the estimate of the influence of unemployment. In the
case of the population over 55 years of age, the lag of
one year is approximately equal in impact of unemployment
to that of two years. For this population, therefore, we
have retained the lag of two years, which is the same as
that used in the prediction equation for the overall population. Only for the populations aged 10-19 and 35-39 is it
substantially more useful to set the effect of unemployment
on mortality at an optimal lag of three years.

Figures 1-4 are examples of graphic analyses of the
relationship of unemployment to mortality rates. Figures 1, 3, and 4 show the relationships for the age groups
55-64, 65-74, and 75-84 with the two-year lagged effect of
unemployment. In Figures 1, 3, and 4 the mortality rates
are detrended for the secular trends and only the residuals
are plotted. In Figure 2, by contrast, both the mortality
data for the age group 55-64 and the unemployment data are
"detrended" by converting the series to annual changes
(i.e., first differences) and then taking 3-year moving
averages to reduce the random "noise" effects. For the
particular data transformation used in Figure 2 (i.e.,
three-year changes) the three-year lag for the effect of
unemployment appears to show a more precise relation to
mortality than the two-year lag.

Figure 2

GRAPHIC ANALYSIS OF THE RELATION BETWEEN THE
TOTAL MORTALITY RATE OF THE POPULATION AGED 55-64
AND THE EMPLOYMENT RATE,* UNITED STATES, 1909-1976

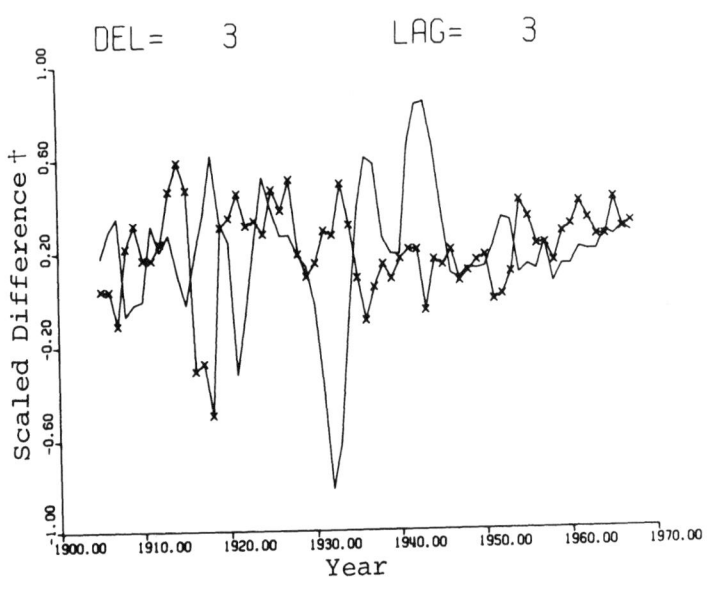

DEL= 3   LAG= 3

—x—x—x—   Total Mortality Rate

_____   U.S. Unemployment Rate,
               Inverted

*Employment Rate = Inverted Unemployment Rate

†Scaled Difference: Both series are scaled for viewing such
that the greatest amplitude from the arithmetic mean of each
series, which is set equal to zero, has been normalized to
+1.00 if positive, or -1.00 if negative.

Del = 3: data transformed to 3-year moving averages of
          annual changes.

Lag = 3: mortality is lagged three years.

Figure 3

GRAPHIC ANALYSIS OF THE RELATION BETWEEN THE
TOTAL MORTALITY RATE OF THE POPULATION AGED 65-74
AND THE EMPLOYMENT RATE,* UNITED STATES, 1909-1976

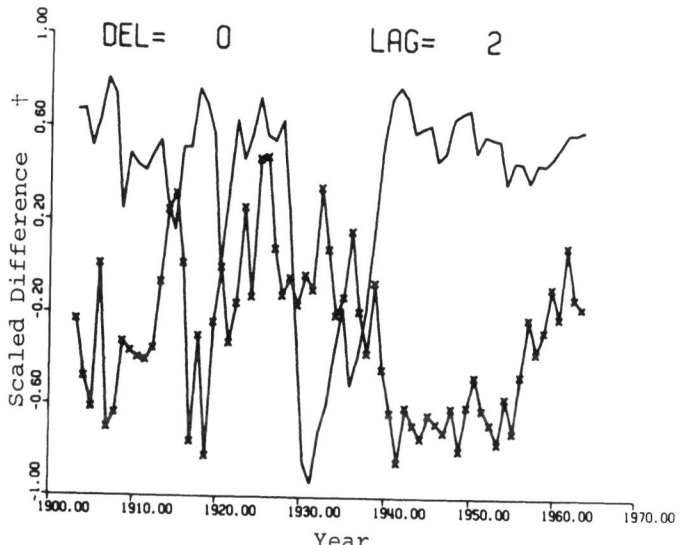

——x—x—x——   Total Mortality Rate

_____   U.S. Unemployment Rate,
Inverted

*Employment Rate = Inverted Unemployment Rate

†Scaled Difference: Both series are scaled for viewing such
that the greatest amplitude from the arithmetic mean of each
series, which is set equal to zero, has been normalized to
+1.00 if positive, or -1.00 if negative.

Del = 0: long-term trends subtracted from the mortality
series.

Lag = 2: mortality is lagged two years.

Figure 4
___

GRAPHIC ANALYSIS OF THE RELATION BETWEEN THE
TOTAL MORTALITY RATE OF THE POPULATION AGED 75-84
AND THE EMPLOYMENT RATE,* UNITED STATES, 1909-1976

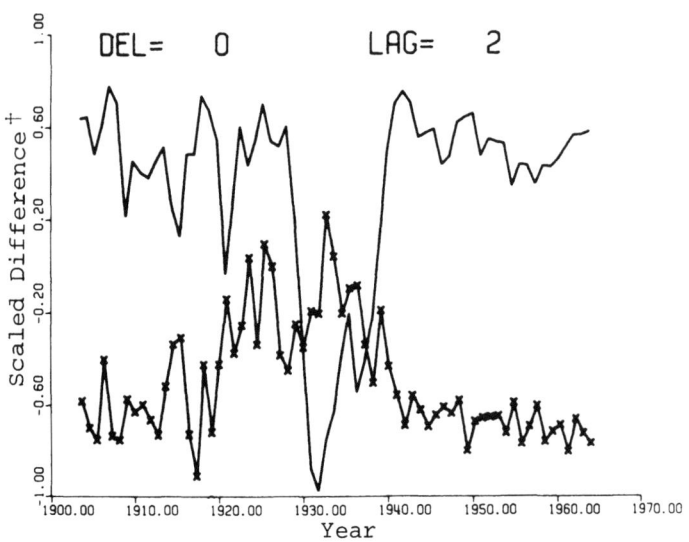

    ―x―x―x―   Total Mortality Rate

    _____   U.S. Unemployment Rate,
                  Inverted

*Employment Rate = Inverted Unemployment Rate

†Scaled Difference: Both series are scaled for viewing such
that the greatest amplitude from the arithmetic mean of each
series, which is set equal to zero, has been normalized to
+1.00 if positive, or -1.00 if negative.

Del = 0: long-term trends subtracted from the mortality
          series.

Lag = 2: mortality is lagged two years.

Conclusions

The central hypotheses specified that several different stresses inherent in the process of economic change influence the mortality rate. These stresses were conceptually organized into three main groups which correspond, for ease of empirical measurement, to: (1) rapid economic growth; (2) substantial loss of economic and social position associated largely with the "recession" phase of the business cycle; and (3) over the long term, the lessening of stress which is influenced by improvements in economic security and medical technology which depend, in turn, on long-term economic growth. Rapid economic growth includes the short-term stresses of: (a) relative deprivation felt by lower socioeconomic groups, especially during the "prosperity" phase of the business cycle; (b) rapid social change, which conflicts with the values, interests, and emotional investments of older persons and others unequipped by job skills or education to cope successfully; and (c) fear stimulated during the "crisis" phase of the business cycle based on the radical and decisive destruction of expectations and aspirations. The stresses of recession can be quite profound and often generate many others either directly or through deprivation of resources with which to deal with other stresses. The cumulative effect influences the mortality rate over the intermediate period of 1-5 years, with a peak or modal effect at approximately two years.

At least the three main elements of the central hypothesis are supported by the data. There are clearly two separately measurable components of the "business cycle" which are shown to be associated with two independent types of stress. Rapid economic change, involving largely the "properity" and "crisis" phases of the cycle, is positively related to mortality within a year's time. The recessional aspect of economic change is associated with elevated mortality rates within 1-5 years, and at a peak lag of two years. Considering the entire period of 1909-76, the most important association of recession to mortality occurs within 1-3 years. The oldest and presumably least healthy populations begin to show elevated mortality rates within a year after the recession, while the population 10-39 years of age, presumably the healthiest, frequently do not show the elevated mortality pattern until three years after the recession. Finally, over the long term, the secular trend of economic growth is inversely related to the mortality rate.

The present analysis, therefore, provides a conclusive test of the short-run as well as the intermediate range impact of the "cyclic" components of economic growth on mortality rates. The fact that the rapid economic growth component of the cycle is strongly positively related to mortality rates synchronously necessarily implies that unemployment rates are often inversely related to mortality rates synchronously. The reason for this is that the lowest periods of unemployment correspond, cyclically, to the "crisis" and "prosperity" phases of rapid economic growth. At the same time, the appropriate relationship of unemployment to mortality rates (without regard to cause) is estimated by observing the mortality rates lagged by at least one year for the population over 55 years of age, and by an average of two to three years for the population as a whole.

The evidence of these two independent effects of the cyclic pattern of economic growth implies that without the appropriate multivariate statistical controls, it may appear to the eye that short- and intermediate-term increases in the mortality rate are causally related to periods of low unemployment (Eyer, 1977). However, if one were to argue that the entire short-run and intermediate reaction of mortality rates to economic changes were based on unemployment alone, one would be faced with the contradiction that unemployment with no lag at all causes mortality to decline while after a year unemployment causes mortality to increase. Thorough, standard, statistical time-series analysis shows instead that the elevated mortality rates which can be seen during periods of rapid economic growth are based on a combination of short-term reactions to the rapid growth phase of economic change and lagged reactions to the previous recessional phase.

These findings, in their broadest sense, indicate that individual stress situations are not randomly distributed through time or space. The pulsating or "cyclic" patterns of economic growth and their aftermath are associated with the "epidemic-like" short-term trends in mortality. The longer-term mortality trends continue to reflect economic growth, although their beneficial impact has been diminishing. These findings can be seen as part of a more general mosaic of research into the social ecology of human stress.

Appendix I

1. Antonovsky, A. "Social Class, Life Expectancy and Over-
    all Mortality." Milbank Memorial Fund Quarterly 45
    (1967): 31-73.

2. Barr, A. "Hospital Admissions and the Social Environ-
    ment." Medical Officer 100 (1958): 351-354.

3. Bergmann, L. and A.S. Yerby. "Low Income and Barriers
    to Use of Health Services." New England Journal of Med-
    icine 278 (1968): 541-546.

4. Borhani, Nemat O. and Thomasina Smith Borkman. Alameda
    County Blood Pressure Study. Berkeley, California:
    State of California, June, 1968.

5. Brockington, F. and S.M. Lempert. The Social Needs of
    the Over-Eighties. Manchester, 1966.

6. Clemmesen, J. and A. Nielsen. "Social Distribution of
    Cancer in Copenhagen, 1943-47." British Journal of Can-
    cer 5 (1951): 159-171.

7. Daric, J. Vital Statistics-Special Reports. Vol. 32,
    No. 10. Washington: U.S. Public Health Service, 1951.

8. Douglas, J.W.B. and J.M. Blomfield. Children Under
    Five. London, 1958.

9. Edwards, F., T. McKeown, and A.G.W. Whitfield. "Contri-
    butions and Demands of Elderly Men." British Journal
    of Preventive Medicine 13 (1959): 59-66.

10. Graham, Saxon, Morton Levin, and Abraham M. Lilenfeld.
    "The Socioeconomic Distribution of Cancer at Various
    Sites in Buffalo, New York: 1948-1952." Cancer 13
    (1960): 80.

11. Guralnick, L. "Selected Family Characteristics and
    Health Measures Reported in the Health Interview Sur-
    vey." P. 6 in Vital and Health Statistics, Publication
    No. 1000. Washington, D.C.: National Center for Health
    Statistics.

12. Hunt, E.P. and E.E. Huyck. "Mortality of White and
    Non-white Infants in Major U.S. Cities." Pp. 23-41 in
    H.E.W. Indicators, Office of Program Analysis.
    Washington, D.C.: Department of Health, Education, and
    Welfare, 1966.

13. Kitagawa, E.M. and P.M. Hauser. "Education Differentials in Mortality by Cause of Death: United States, 1960." Demography 5 (1968): 318-353.

14. Logan, W.P.D. "Social Class Variations in Mortality." British Journal of Preventive Social Medicine 8 (1954): 128-137.

15. Marr, J.W., E.B. Hope, L.D. Stevenson, and A.M. Thompson. "Consumption of Milk and Vitamin Concentrates by Pregnant Women in Aberdeen." Proceedings of the Nutrition Society 14 (1955): 7.

16. Morris, J.N. Uses of Epidemiology. Edinburgh, 1964.

17. Registrar General's Decennial Supplement England and Wales, 1921, Part II, Occupational Mortality, Fertility and Infant Mortality, London: H.M.S.O., 1927.

18. Susser, M.W. and W. Watson. Chapter 4 in Sociology in Medicine (2nd ed.). New York: Oxford University Press, 1971.

19. Sydenstricker, E. "Economic Status and the Incidence of Illness." Hagerstown Morbidity Studies, No. 10. U.S. Public Health Report 44 (1929): 1821-1833.

20. Young, M. "Variation in Mortality from Cancer of Different Parts of the Body in Groups of Men of Different Social Status." Journal of Hygiene (London) 25 (1926): 209-217.

Appendix II

1. Adelstein, A.M., D.Y. Dunhan, Z.A. Stein, and M.W. Susser. "The Epidemiology of Mental Illness in an English City." Social Psychiatry 3 (1968): 47-59.

2. Brooke, E.M. "National Statistics in the Epidemiology of Mental Health." Journal of Mental Science 105 (1959): 893-908.

3. Cahalan, D., I.H. Cisin, and H.M. Crossley. American Drinking Practices: A National Survey of Drinking Behavior and Attitudes. New Brunswick: Rutgers Center for Alcohol Studies, 1969.

4. Clark, R.E. "The Relationship of Schizophrenia to Occupational Income and Prestige." American Sociological Review 13 (1948): 325-330.

5. Clark, R.E. "Psychoses, Income and Occupational Prestige: Schizophrenia in American Cities." American Journal of Sociology 54 (1949): 433-440.

6. Colcord, J.C. Broken Homes. New York: Russell Sage Foundation, 1919.

7. Dooghie, Gilbert. "Premarital Conception with Married Couples According to Socio-Professional Status." Journal of Marriage and the Family 80: 124-128.

8. Empey, Lamar T. and Maynard L. Erickson. "Hidden Delinquency and Social Status." Social Forces 44 (June, 1966): 546-554.

9. Faris, R.E.L. and H.W. Dunham. Mental Disorders in Urban Areas: An Ecological Study of Schizophrenia and Other Psychoses. New York, 1960.

10. Goode, William J. Women in Divorce. New York: Free Press, 1965.

11. Goode, William J. "Marital Satisfaction and Instability: A Cross-cultural Class Analysis of Divorce Rates." International Social Science Journal 14, 3 (1962): 507-526.

12. Gurin, G., J. Veroff, and S. Feld. Americans View Their Mental Health. Monograph, Series 4. New York: Joint Commission on Mental Illness and Health.

13. Hardt, Robert H.   "Delinquency and Social Class: Bad Kids or Good Cops."   Pp. 132-145 in Irwin Deutscher and Elizabeth J. Thompson, eds., Among the People: Encounters with the Poor.   New York: Basic Books, 1968.

14. Hare, E.H.   "Mental Illness and Social Class in Bristol."   British Journal of Preventive and Social Medicine 102 (1956): 349-357.

15. Hillman, Karen G.   "Marital Instability and Its Relation to Education, Income and Occupation: An Analysis Based on Census Data."   Pp. 603-608 in R.F. Winch, et al., eds.   Selected Studies in Marriage and the Family (rev. ed.).   New York: Holt, 1962.

16. Hollingshead, August B. and F.C. Redlich.   Social Class and Mental Illness.   New York, 1958.

17. Innes, G. and G.A. Sharp.   "A Study of Psychiatric Patients in North-East Scotland."   Journal of Mental Science 108 (1922): 447-456.

18. Jaco, E.G.   The Social Epidemiology of Mental Disorders: A Psychiatric Study of Texas.   New York: Russell Sage Foundation, 1960.

19. Kephart, William M. and Thomas P. Monahan.   "Desertion and Divorce in Philadelphia."   American Sociological Review 17 (December, 1952): 719-720.

20. Leighton, D.C., J.S. Harding, D.B. Macklin, A.M. MacMillan, and A.H. Leighton.   The Character of Danger: Psychiatric Symptoms in Selected Communities. Stirling County Study 3.   New York: Basic Books, 1963.

21. Pasamanick, B., ed.   "Epidemiology of Mental Disorder." American Association for the Advancement of Science. Publication No. 60.   Washington, D.C., 1959.

22. Srole, L., T.S. Langner, S.T. Michael, M.K. Opler, and T.A.C. Rennie.   Mental Health in the Metropolis: The Midtown Manhattan Study.   New York, 1962.

23. Stein, L.   "Social Class' Gradient in Schizophrenia." British Journal of Preventive and Social Medicine 11 (1957): 181-195.

24. Susser, Mervyn W.   Community Psychiatry: Epidemiological and Social Themes.   New York, 1968.

25. Tietze, C., P.V. Lemkau, and M.M. Cooper. "Schizophrenia, Manic-Depressive Psychosis and Social Economic Status." <u>American Journal of Sociology</u> 47 (1941): 167-175.

26. Van Nye, F., James F. Short, Jr., and V.J. Olson. "Socioeconomic Status and Delinquent Behavior." <u>American Journal of Sociology</u> 63 (January, 1958): 381-389.

Appendix III

1. Abernathy, W.J. and E.L. Schrems. "Distance and Health Services: Issues of Utilization and Facility Choice for Demographic Strata." Research Paper No. 19. Stanford University: Graduate School of Business, 1971.

2. Andersen, R. A Behavioral Model of Families' Use of Health Services. Research Series, No. 25, Center for Health Administration Studies. Chicago: University of Chicago Press, 1968.

3. Andersen, R. and O.W. Anderson. A Decade of Health Services. Chicago: University of Chicago Press, 1967.

4. Andersen, R. and L. Benham. "Factors Affecting the Relationship Between Family Income and Medical Care Consumption." In H.E. Klarman, ed. Empirical Studies in Health Economics. Baltimore: The Johns Hopkins Press, 1970.

5. Andersen, R., et al. Medical Care Use in Sweden and the United States--A Comparative Analysis of Systems and Behavior. Research Series No. 27. Center for Health Administration Studies. Chicago: University of Chicago Press, 1970.

6. Andersen, R., et al. "Perceptions of and Response to Symptoms of Illness in Sweden and the United States." Medical Care 6 (January-February, 1968): 18-31.

7. Anderson, J.G. "Demographic Factors Affecting Health Services Utilization: A Causal Model." Unpublished manuscript. Purdue University: Department of Sociology, 1972.

8. Anderson, O.W. and R. Andersen. "Patterns of Use of Health Services." In H. Freeman, et al., eds. Handbook of Medical Sociology. Englewood Cliffs, New Jersey: Prentice-Hall, 1972.

9. Anderson, O.W., et al. Changes in Family Medical Care Expenditures and Voluntary Health Insurance. Cambridge: Harvard University Press, 1963.

10. Antonovsky, A. and R. Katz. "The Model Dental Patient: An Empirical Study of Preventive Health Behavior." Social Science and Medicine 4 (November, 1970): 267-280.

11. Bergner, L. and A. Yerby. "Low Income and Barriers to Use of Health Services." New England Journal of Medicine 278 (March 7, 1968): 541-546.

12. Bice, T.W. "Medical Care for the Disadvantaged: Report on a Survey of Use of Medical Services in the Baltimore Standard Metropolitan Statistical Area 1968-1969." Final report of research conducted under Contract Number HSM 110 69 203, NCHSRD, 1971.

13. Bice, T.W. and R.L. Eichhorn. "Socioeconomic Status and Use of Physicians' Services: A Reconsideration." Medical Care 12 (May-June, 1972): 261-271.

14. Bice, T.W., et al. "Economic Class and Use of Physicians' Services." Unpublished manuscript. Johns Hopkins University: Department of Medical Care and Hospitals, 1971.

15. Bashshur, R.L., et al. "Some Ecological Differentials in the Use of Medical Services." Health Services Research 6 (Spring, 1971): 61-75.

16. Darsky, B.J., et al. Comprehensive Medical Services Under Voluntary Health Insurance: A Study of Windsor Medical Services. Cambridge: Harvard University Press.

17. Densen, P.M., et al. "Concerning High and Low Utilizers of Services on Medical Care Plan, and the Persistence of Utilization Levels over a Three-Year Period." Milbank Memorial Fund Quarterly 37 (July, 1959): 217-250.

18. Dodge, W.F., et al. "Patterns of Maternal Desires for Child Health Care." American Journal of Public Health 60 (August, 1970): 1421-1429.

19. Durbin, R.L. and G. Antelman. "A Study of the Effects of Selected Variables on Hospital Utilization." Hospital Management 98 (August, 1964): 57-60.

20. Feldstein, P.J. "Research on the Demand for Health Services." Milbank Memorial Fund Quarterly 44 (July, 1966): 128-162.

21. Fink, R., et al. "The Reluctant Participant in Breast Cancer Screening Programs." Public Health Reports 83 (June, 1968): 479-490.

22. Fitzpatrick, T.B., et al. "Character and Effective-
    ness of Hospital Use." In W.J. McNerney, et al.
    Hospital and Medical Economics. Chicago: Hospital
    Research and Educational Trust, 1962.

23. Klem, M.C. "Physician Services Received in an Urban
    Community in Relation to Health Insurance Coverage."
    American Journal of Public Health 55 (November, 1965):
    1699-1716.

24. Kriesberg, L. "The Relationship Between Socio-economic
    Rank and Behavior." Social Problems 10 (Spring, 1963):
    334-352.

25. Ludwig, E.G. and G. Gibson. "Self Perception of Sick-
    ness and the Seeking of Medical Care." Journal of
    Health and Social Behavior 10 (June, 1969): 125-132.

26. Muller, C. "Income and the Receipt of Medical Care."
    American Journal of Public Health 55 (April, 1965):
    510-521.

27. National Center for Health Statistics. Age Patterns
    in Medical Care, Illness, and Disability: United
    States -- July 1963-June 1965. Series 10, No. 32.
    Washington, 1966.

28. National Center for Health Statistics. Children and
    Youth -- Selected Health Characteristics: United
    States -- 1958 and 1968. Series 10, No. 62. Washing-
    ton, 1971.

29. National Center for Health Statistics. Current Esti-
    mates from the Health Interview Survey: United
    States -- July 1964. Series 10, No. 13. Washington,
    1964.

30. National Center for Health Statistics. Differentials
    in Health Characteristics by Color: United States --
    July 1965-June 1967. Series 10, No. 56. Washington,
    1969.

31. National Center for Health Statistics. Family Income
    in Relation to Selected Health Characteristics.
    Series 10, No. 2. Washington, 1963.

32. National Center for Health Statistics. Family Use of
    Health Services: United States -- July 1963-June 1964.
    Series 10, No. 55. Washington, 1969.

33. National Center for Health Statistics. Hospital Discharges and Length of Stay: Short-Stay Hospitals: United States -- July 1963-June 1964. Series 10, No. 30. Washington, 1966.

34. National Center for Health Statistics. Medical Care, Health Status, and Family Income: United States -- 1963. Series 10, No. 9. Washington, 1964.

35. National Center for Health Statistics. Personal Health Expenses -- Per Capital Annual Expenses: United States -- July-December 1962. Series 10, No. 27. Washington, 1966.

36. National Center for Health Statistics. Persons Hospitalized by Number of Hospital Episodes and Days in a Year: United States -- July 1960-June 1962. Series 10, No. 20. Washington, 1965.

37. National Center for Health Statistics. Persons Hospitalized by Number of Hospital Illness Episodes and Days in a Year: United States -- July 1965-June 1966. Series 10, No. 50. Washington, 1969.

38. National Center for Health Statistics. Physician Visits -- Interval of Visits and Children's Routine Checkup: United States -- July 1963-June 1964. Series 10, No. 19. Washington, 1965.

39. National Center for Health Statistics. Volume of Dental Visits: United States -- July 1963-June 1964. Series 10, No. 23. Washington, 1965.

40. National Center for Health Statistics. Volume of Physician Visits: United States -- July 1966-June 1967. Series 10, No. 49. Washington, 1968.

41. Purola, T., et al. The Utilization of Medical Services and Its Relationship to Morbidity, Health Resources and Social Factors. Helsinki: Research Institute for Social Security, 1968.

42. Richardson, A.M., et al. "Use of Medical Resources by SPANCOS: II. Social Factors and Medical Care Experience." Milbank Memorial Fund Quarterly 45 (January, 1967): 61-75.

43. Richardson, W.C. "Measuring the Urban Poor's Use of Physicians' Services in Response to Illness Episodes." Medical Care 8 (March-April, 1970): 132-142.

44. Richardson, W.C. "Poverty, Illness and Use of Health Services in the United States." Hospital 43 (July 1, 1969): 34-40.

45. Ross, J.A. "Social Class and Medical Care." Journal of Health and Human Behavior 4 (Spring, 1962): 35-40.

46. Sparer, G. and L. Sparer. "Differential Patterns of Poverty and Health Care Utilization in Eight Urban Areas." Paper presented at the meetings of the American Association for Public Opinion Research. Pasadena, California, May 22, 1971.

47. U.S. Public Health Service. Population Characteristics and Participation in the Poliomyelitis Vaccination Program. PHS No. 722. Washington, D.C.: U.S. Government Printing Office, 1960.

48. U.S. Public Health Service. Proceedings of a Conference on Conceptual Issues in the Analysis of Medical Care Utilization Behavior. Conference sponsored by Kaiser Foundation Hospitals and National Center for Health Services Research and Development. Portland, Oregon, October, 1969.

49. White, E.L. "A Graphic Presentation on Age and Income Differentials in Selected Aspects of Morbidity, Disability, and Utilization of Health Services." Inquiry 5 (March, 1968): 18-30.

50. Winkelstein, W., Jr. and S. Graham. "Factors in Participation in the 1954 Poliomyelitis Vaccine Field Trials, Erie County, New York." American Journal of Public Health 49 (November, 1959): 1454-1466.

51. Wirick, G.C. "A Multiple Equation Model of Demand for Health Care." Health Services Research 1 (Winter, 1966): 301-346.

Appendix IV

1. Brenner, M. Harvey. "Cardiovascular-Renal Disease Mortality and Economic Instability in the United States." Paper presented at the annual meeting of the American Public Health Association, 1973.

2. Brenner, M. Harvey. "Economic Changes and Heart Disease Mortality." American Journal of Public Health 61 (March, 1971): 606-611.

3. Brenner, M. Harvey. "Economic Instability and Mental Hospitalization in the United States, 1922-1968: An Issue of Primary Prevention in Severe Mental Disorders." Paper presented at the Annual Meeting of the American Public Health Association, 1973.

4. Brenner, M. Harvey. "Effects of the Economy on Criminal Behavior and the Administration of Criminal Justice in the United States, Canada, England and Wales, and Scotland." In Economic Crises and Crime: Correlations Between the State of the Economy, Deviance and the Control of Deviance. Rome, Italy: United Nations Social Defense Research Institute, 1976.

5. Brenner, M. Harvey. "Fetal, Infant, and Maternal Mortality During Periods of Economic Instability." International Journal of Health Services 3, 1974.

6. Brenner, M. Harvey. Mental Illness and the Economy. Cambridge, Massachusetts: Harvard University Press, 1973.

7. Brenner, M. Harvey. Time Series Analysis of the Relationships Between Selected Economic and Social Indicators. 2 Volumes. Springfield, Virginia: National Technical Information Service, March, 1971.

8. Brenner, M. Harvey. "Trends in Alcohol Consumption and Associated Illnesses." American Journal of Public Health 65, December, 1975.

9. Dayton, Neil A. New Facts on Mental Disorders. Springfield, Illinois: Charles C. Thomas, 1940.

10. Frederiksen, H. "Dynamic Equilibrium of Economics to Demographic Transition." Economic Development and Cultural Change 14, April, 1966.

11. Frederiksen, H. "Feedbacks in Economic and Demographic Transition." Science 166, November, 1969.

12. Goldscheider, Calvin. "The Mortality Revolution." Chapter 5 in Population, Modernization, and Social Structure. Boston: Little, Brown and Company, 1971.

13. Henry, A.F. and T.F. Short, Jr. Suicide and Homicide. Glencoe, Illinois: Free Press, 1954.

14. MacMahon, Brian, S. Johnson, and T.F. Pugh. "Relation of Suicide to Social Conditions." U.S. Public Health Reports 78: 285-293.

15. McKeown, Thomas. "A Sociological Approach to the History of Medicine." Chapter 2 in Gordon McLachlan and Thomas McKeown, eds., Medical History and Medical Care. London: Oxford University Press, 1971.

16. Pugh, Thomas F. and Brian MacMahon. Epidemiological Findings in United States Mental Hospital Data. Boston: Little, Brown and Company, 1962.

17. United Nations. The Situation and Recent Trends of Mortality in the World. Population Bulletin No. 6, Table IV. 1., 1963.

18. United Nations. Department of Economic and Social Affairs. The Determinants and Consequences of Population Trends: New Summary of Findings on Interaction of Demographic, Economic and Social Factors. Population Studies, No. 50. 2 Volumes. New York: United Nations, 1973.

Appendix V

Data Derivations and Sources

1. Welfare Expenditures

    The variable is defined as:

    $$\frac{\text{Welfare Expenditures}}{\text{General Expenditures}} \times 100$$

    where Welfare Expenditures are defined as Total Social
    Welfare Expenditures less Education Expenditures, and
    General Expenditures are defined as Total Government
    Expenditures summed for Federal, State, and Local
    governments.

    The data for General Expenditures for the years 1909-
    1970* are found in (1), Part 2, Series Y533-566, #534,
    p.1120. For the years 1971-76, they are found in (2),
    Table 499, p. 317.**

    The data for Welfare Expenditures for the years 1909-
    1970 are found in (1), Part 1, Series H1-31 and H32-
    47, pp. 340-341. For the years 1971-76, they are found
    in (2), Table 499, p. 317.**

    The Total Social Welfare Expenditure data are linearly
    interpolated for the years 1914-1928. The General
    Expenditure data are interpolated for the years 1915-
    26, 1928-31, 1933, 1935, 1937, 1939, 1941, 1943, 1945,
    1947, 1949, and 1951.

2. Per Capita Personal Income

    The variable is defined as:

    Per capita personal income in constant 1972 dollars

    The data for the years 1975 and 1976 are found in (2),
    Table 694, p. 431. For the years 1929-74, they are
    found in (4), Table 8.8, p. 313. The data for the
    years 1909-28 are calculated as follows:

    $$\frac{\text{Disposable Personal Income}}{\substack{\text{Implicit Price Deflator} \\ \text{for 1929***}}} \times \frac{1}{\text{Population}}$$

---

* Alaska and Hawaii are first included in 1960
** Data for 1976 are preliminary
***Implicit Price Deflator for 1929 is .3287

The data for disposable personal income are found in
(3), Series A37-A47, p.188. Values are interpolated for
the years 1910-13 and 1915-18. The implicit price deflator for 1929 in 1972 dollars is found in (4). The
population data are interpolated from the decennial
census.

3. Unemployment Rate

The variable is defined as:

Number of persons unemployed
Number of persons in the
civilian labor force

where unemployed persons are persons 16 years old and
over, who did not work during the survey week, who were
seeking work, who were available for work except for
temporary illness, or who were waiting to be called
back to a job after being laid off.

The data for the years 1909-74 are found in (5), Table
60, p. 146. For the years 1975 and 1976, they are
found in (2), Table 642, p. 395.

4. Sources

1. U. S. Bureau of the Census. Historical Statistics
    of the United States, Colonial Times to 1970,
    Bicentennial Edition, Parts 1 and 2,
    Washington, D. C., 1975.

2. U. S. Bureau of the Census. Statistical Abstract
    of the United States: 1977.(98th edition)
    Washington, D. C., 1977.

3. U. S. Department of Commerce. Long Term Economic
    Growth: 1860-1970. Washington, D. C., 1973.

4. U. S. Department of Commerce, Office of Business
    Statistics. The National Income and Product
    Accounts of the United States, 1929-74:
    Statistical Tables. Washington, D. C., 1976.

5. U. S. Department of Labor, Bureau of Labor Stat-
    istics. Handbook of Labor Statistics, 1975—
    Reference Edition. Washington, D. C., 1977.

Note

The author gratefully acknowledges support for this research from the National Institute of Mental Health, Center for studies of Metropolitan Problems, under grant No. MH 26154, entitled Economic Change and Social Pathologies in Urban Areas.

References

Adelman, Irma. "An Econometric Analysis of Population Growth." American Economic Review 53 (June 1963): 314-339.

Alexander, Franz. Psychosomatic Medicine: Its Principles and Applications. New York: Norton, 1950.

Anderson, Odin W. Health Care: Can There be Equity? The United States, Sweden, and England. New York: Wiley Interscience, 1972.

Bales, R.F. "Adaptive and Integrative Changes as Sources of Strain in Social Systems." In A. Paul Hare, E.F. Borgatta and Robert F. Bales, eds. Small Groups: Studies in Social Interaction. New York: Alfred A. Knopf, 1966.

Blau, Peter M. Exchange and Power in Social Life. New York: John Wiley and Sons, 1964.

Brenner, M. Harvey. Estimating the Social Costs of National Economic Policy: Implications for Mental and Physical Health, and Criminal Aggression. Joint Economic Committee of the U.S. Congress, Washington, D.C., 1976.

Brenner, M. Harvey. "Influence of the Social Environment on Psychopathology: The Historical Perspective," in J.E. Barrett, R.M. Rose, G.L. Klerman, eds., Stress and Mental Disorder, New York: Raven Press (forthcoming), 1979. Revised paper entitled "Impact of Social and Industrial Changes in Psychopathology: A View of Stress from the Standpoint of Macro Societal Trends," in Lennart Levi, ed., Society, Stress, and Disease, London: Oxford University Press (forthcoming), 1979.

Burgess, Robert L., and Don Bushell, Jr. Behavioral Sociology: The Experimental Analysis of Social Process. New York: Columbia University Press, 1969.

Caplan, Bert., John Cassel, and Susan Gore. "Social Support and Health." Medical Care, 15 Supplement (1977): 47-58.

Cassel, John. "Physical Illness in Response to Stress." Pp. 189-209 in Sol Levine and Norman A. Scotch, eds., Social Stress. Chicago: Aldine Publishing Co., 1970.

Cochrane, Donald and Guy H. Orcutt. "Application of Least Squares Regression to Relationships Containing Auto-Correlated Error Terms." Journal of the American Statistical Association 44 (March, 1949): 32-61.

Dodge, D.L., and W.T. Martin. Social Stress and Chronic Illness, Notre Dame, Ind.: University of Notre Dame Press, 1970.

Durbin, J., and G.S. Watson. "Testing for Serial Correlation in Least Squares Regression." pts. I and II. Biometrika, 1950, 1951.

Durkheim, Emile. Suicide: A Study in Sociology. Trans. by John A. Spaulding and George Simpson, edited with an introduction by G. Simpson. Glencoe: Free Press, 1951. (First published in Paris: F. Alcan: 1897)

Eyer, J. "Prosperity as a Cause of Death." International Journal of Health Services, 7 (1977): 125-150.

Frederiksen, H. "Feedbacks in Economic and Demographic Transition." Science 166 (November, 1969): 837-847.

Gersten, J.C., T.S. Langner, J.G. Eisenberg, and L. Orzeck. "Child Behavior and Life Events: Undesirable Change or Change per se?" Pp. 159-170 in B.S. Dohrenwend and B.P. Dohrenwend, eds., Stressful Life Events: Their Nature and Effects. New York: Wiley - Interscience, 1974.

Gross, Edward. "Work Organization, and Stress." In Sol Levine and Norman A. Scotch, eds., Social Stress. Chicago: Aldine Press, 1970.

Henry, Andrew F., and James F. Short. Suicide and Homicide. Glencoe: Free Press, 1954.

Holmes, T.H. and M.N. Masuda. "Life Change and Illness Susceptibility." Pp. 45-79 in B.S. Dohrenwend and B.P. Dohrenwend, eds., Stressful Life Events: Their Nature and Effects. New York: Wiley - Interscience, 1974.

Holmes, T.H. and R.H. Rahe. "The Social Readjustment Rating Scale." Journal of Psychosomatic Research 11 (1967): 213-218.

Homans, George C. Social Behavior: Its Elementary Forms. New York: Harcourt, Brace, and World, 1961.

Jackson, Elton F. "Status Consistency and Symptoms of Stress." American Sociological Review 27 (1962): 469-480.

Johns, Edward A. The Sociology of Organizational Change. London: Oxford University Press, 1973.

Keyfitz, Nathan. "Demographic Methods and Their Application in the Social and Health Sciences." In this volume.

Kleiner, Robert T. and Seymour Parker. "Goal Striving, Social Status and Mental Disorder: A Research Review." American Sociological Review 28 (April, 1963): 189-202.

Lave, Lester B. and Eugene P. Seskin. Air Pollution and Human Health. Baltimore: The Johns Hopkins Press for Resources for the Future, 1977.

Lenski, Gerhard E. "Status Crystalization: A Non-Vertical Dimension of Social Status." American Sociological Review 19 (1954): 405-413.

Levi, Lennart. "Stress and Distress in Response to Psychosocial Stimuli." Acta Med. Scand., 191 Supplement 528. (Simultaneously published in book form by Pergamon Press, Oxford, 1972.)

Lilienfeld, A.M. and A.J. Gifford, eds. Chronic Diseases and Public Health. Baltimore: Johns Hopkins Press, 1966.

Merton, Robert K. Social Theory and Social Structure. Glencoe: The Free Press, 1957, Chapter IV.

Meyer, Adolf. "The Life Chart and the Obligation of Specifying Positive Data in Psychopathological Diagnosis." Pp. 52-56, in E. Winters, ed., The Collected Papers of Adolf Meyer, Volume III, Medical Teaching. Baltimore: The Johns Hopkins University Press, 1951.

Mills, Theodore M. Group Transformation: An Analysis of a Learning Group. Englewood Cliffs: Prentice Hall, 1964, Chapter V, "Toward a Conception of the Life Cycle of Groups."

Moss, G.E. Illness, Stress, and Social Interaction. New York: John Wiley, 1973.

Mueller, Daniel P., Daniel W. Edwards, and Richard M. Yarvis. "Stressful Life Events and Psychiatric Symptomatology: Change or Undesirability?" Journal of Health and Social Behavior 18 (September, 1977): 307-317.

Parsons, Talcott. The Social System. Glencoe: The Free Press, 1951, Chapter VII.

Paykel, E.S. "Recent Life Events and Clinical Depression." Pp. 134-163 in E.K. Eric Gunderson and R.H. Rahe, eds., Life Stress and Illness. Springfield, Illinois: Charles C. Thomas, 1974.

Preston, Samuel. Mortality Patterns in National Populations. New York: Academic Press, 1976, Chapter IV.

Rahe, R.H., M. Meyer, M. Smith, G. Kjaer, and T.H. Holmes. "Social Stress and Illness Onset." Journal of Psychosomatic Research 8 (1964): 35-44.

Rogers, Everett M. Diffusion of Innovations. New York: Free Press, 1962.

Schmidt, Peter and Roger N. Wand. "The Almon Lag Technique and the Monetary Versus Fiscal Policy." Journal of the American Statistical Association 68 (March, 1973): 11-15.

Selye, Hans. The Stress of Life. New York: McGraw Hill Book Company, 1956.

Slater, Philip E. "Role Differentiation in Small Groups."
In A. Paul Hare, E.F. Borgatta and Robert F. Bales,
eds., Small Groups: Studies in Social Interaction.
New York: Alfred A. Knopf, 1966.

Smelser, Neil J. "Mechanisms of Change and Adjustment to
Change." Pp. 32-54, in Bert F. Hoselitz and Wilbert
E. Moore, eds., Industrialization and Society. The
Hague: UNESCO and Mouton, 1963.

Starbuck, William H. "Organizational Growth and Development." In James G. March, Handbook of Organizations.
Chicago: Rand McNally and Company, 1965.

U. S. Social Security Administration, Office of Research and
Statistics. Social Security Programs Throughout the
World: 1977. Research Report No. 50.
Washington, 1978.

Webster's Third New International Dictionary of the English
Language Unabridged, 1971.

World Bank. World Development Report, 1978. Washington,
D.C.: The International Bank for Reconstruction and
Development of the World Bank, August, 1978.

Jude Thomas May, Katherine Knoop Parry,
Mary L. Durham, Peter Kong-ming New

3. Institutional Structure and Process in Health Services Innovation: The Reform Strategy of the Neighborhood Health Center Program

Introduction

The term "neighborhood (or community) health center" (NHC) identifies federally-funded, comprehensive, primary health care programs which provide a wide range of medically-related services for low-income populations throughout the United States. There are approximately 420 of these centers located in both rural and urban settings. In fiscal year (FY) 1977, approximately 11.7 million medical encounters were recorded at these NHC's, which provide the principal source of health care for over 3.3 million people. These centers are administered by local organizations and supported through the authority of Section 330 of the Public Health Service Act. The budget for FY 1977 was slightly over 215 million dollars, and an increase of 32 million dollars is anticipated for FY 1978. This increase, and the projected expansion of the number of new NHC's, reflects the emphasis which the current administration has placed on the health center as an effective model for delivering preventive health services, particularly among the poor.

The existing NHC program was initiated in 1965 by the Office of Economic Opportunity (OEO). Project grants were awarded by that agency to local health institutions, such as medical schools, hospitals, and health boards, to initiate and administer NHC programs. Although the first projects were funded on a research and demonstration basis, the

The authors wish to acknowledge the financial support provided through the National Association of Community Health Centers, Inc., and the encouragement of Mr. L. Jerome Ashford, Executive Director, and Dr. Danny Davis, President.

program was expanded rapidly, and, by January of 1968, a total of 41 programs had been funded at an approximate annual
cost of 60 million dollars. The program continued to expand
in the following years, and, in 1971-72, the authority for
the NHC's was transferred to the Public Health Service (PHS)
in the Department of Health, Education and Welfare (D/HEW)
(May, et al., 1976).

The NHC program was initially conceived as an innovative
response to the growing evidence of the need for health services for the poor. Beyond this service function, however,
the originators of the program considered it an effective
mechanism for "reforming" the existing health care system.
They reasoned that the existing system, typified by increasing specialization in medicine, overemphasis on complex ter-
tiary care, and fragmentation of services, was partially responsible for the poor medical care received by low-income
populations. Their goal was to demonstrate a new model of
health services delivery which, by example, would point up
the shortcomings of these trends. In turn, this model would
document the importance of a health care system which was
comprehensive and family/neighborhood centered. Finally, the
process of developing and demonstrating this model, in joint
sponsorship with local health organizations, would provide
the vehicle for reforming those institutions.

The development of the goals and strategy to achieve
these changes may best be understood from a perspective which
focuses on (a) the process of institutional change, and
(b) the activities and functions of the organization.

Social problems, according to Morse, arise because of a
perceived "strain" in the social system, and require institutional change for their resolution (Morse, 1969). The process of institutional change includes several phases: problem recognition, problem formulation, and the operationalization of change through an appropriate institution. Morse
notes that the initiation of change must occur in an institution which is sufficiently flexible to act in a manner
free from constraint. This may be achieved through the
"adaptation of workable institutional arrangements,... or the
invention of new ones." In turn, the innovation may be operationalized most effectively at the local level by institutions which are characterized by similar concerns and interests (Morse, 1969).

The activities of an organization are directed toward
particular functions, which, in turn, provide a means to

understand and typify that organization. These functions
may be directed toward (a) achieving specific goals, or
(b) maintaining the existence of the organizational system.
The functions of an organization may be oriented simultaneously to specific goals and system maintenance. Furthermore,
an organization may alter its activities and functions over
time (Morse, 1969).

Purpose of the Paper

This paper will analyze the process of developing a
health services innovation. The strategy and tactics of reform within the framework of institutional change will be
described, beginning with problem definition and continuing
through the operationalization of change. We will analyze
the goals of the NHC program as well as those of the local
health institutions which sponsored specific projects, con-
tending that significant differences in orientation existed.

We will argue that the initial NHC program emphasized
activities which served goal-oriented functions. As the
program expanded, increasing emphasis was placed on system
maintenance functions, which became an overriding concern
after 1969 because of changes in the social and political
milieu. Although the budget for the program continued to
increase and the number of NHC's increased, the goal of reforming health institutions was no longer viable.

The Data

The study is based on in-depth, focused interviews with
79 key individuals who were associated with the NHC program
sponsored by the OEO and the PHS.[1] The respondents included
officials at the national level (N = 44), as well as project
directors and administrators associated with various programs
throughout the country (N = 35).[2] Respondents for the study
included all officials who had held key positions in the NHC
program office of the OEO. Local project officials were selected to include the following: directors of "early" and
"later" projects; physicians and non-physicians; directors
from large and small projects; and directors from projects
in different regions of the country. The interviews were
arranged and completed during the period 1974-77.[3] The study
also included a search of relevant documents, such as the
quarterly status reports prepared within the OEO health office beginning in 1965.

The Strategy and Tactics of Institutional Change

Identification of the Problem

The general perspective which guided the formulation of programs within OEO during the initial phase depicted the poor as a population manipulated by a wide range of social forces which ultimately were responsible for a particular life style. These forces functioned as a reinforcing "cycle" narrowing the opportunities of the poor. The result was a new form of poverty, characterized by the interrelationship of social forces in a highly complex society.

Integral to this viewpoint was the judgment that the existing system of social welfare programs, whether private or public, was inadequate because it was fragmented, insensitive, and unable to respond to the basic nature and characteristics of this new poverty. In point of fact, it was argued, these programs were often a part of the problem. A more appropriate response, critics contended, must be predicated on an innovative, multi-faceted program of human services sponsored by the federal government.

Health care was not a program priority within OEO during the first months of the organization. For example, the first Director of the agency, Sargent Shriver, recalled that "at the very beginning,... health services for the poor was not one of the principal concentrations for my attention." (Shriver, 1976) The administration of the agency assumed that this type of activity was being carried out by other organizations within the government, specifically the PHS. However, it soon became evident, through early data from other programs, that levels of physical impairment and illness among poverty program participants were a major problem.

> Through the Job Corps and Neighborhood Youth Corps they found young men whose teeth were all gone already at 18, who had unrepaired hernias and a whole variety of other lesions... They found themselves laying out large sums of money to pay the private sector for the repair of these things in a catch-up kind of way. (Gibson, 1974)

Almost simultaneously, Mr. Shriver became acquainted with the extent of existing government health care programs for the poor and the orientation of the sponsoring agencies. A joint meeting with key officials from the PHS was arranged to identify areas of support and cooperation. According to one participant, the meeting convinced Mr. Shriver that the

PHS could not be counted upon as a source of programmatic support.

> When the Public Health Service [representatives] got through stating what their plans were, Mr. Shriver reacted very angrily and said it was the same old tired set of programs that they had been peddling for a number of years, and that he was looking for much more innovation and commitment than what he found.[4]

Mr. Shriver's assessment of the existing federal programs was similar to the evaluation of some critics of the broader health care delivery system. Specifically, these critics noted that the distribution of private health professionals was disproportionately sparse in urban ghettos, forcing the poor to rely for care on teaching hospital clinics, emergency rooms, and public health clinics, when such facilities were available. In each of these settings, the nature and quality of health care were marginal at best; and the description of one prominent medical care official found wide currency as an apt evaluation: "Poor people are forced to barter their dignity for health care." (Schorr and English, 1968) To a large extent, critics argued, this resulted from the fact that most of the health institutions responsible for the care of the poor had other priorities, such as teaching and research.

Formulation of the Problem

From the earliest months of the organization of the agency, there were individuals within OEO who had expertise in health. Their activities, however, were largely confined to the operations of more traditional health-related activities which were supportive of other programs, such as medical examinations for participants in poverty projects. These individuals, specifically Dr. Julius Richmond (serving at the time as Director of Project Head Start), Lisbeth Bamberger Schorr [in the Office of Research and Demonstration, Community Action Program (CAP)] , and Dr. Sanford Kravitz (Director of the Office of Research and Demonstration, CAP), generally agreed with the criticisms of the existing health care delivery system noted above.

The first applications for support of health services programs which came into OEO in the Spring of 1965 were small requests for projects which would supplement existing service programs. In conversations with Drs. Richmond and Kravitz, Ms. Schorr determined that:

It would be a big mistake for OEO to be spending any
substantial amounts of funds on health services deliv-
ered through the traditional delivery system. (Schorr,
1975)

Any attempt to resolve the problem, they decided, had to be
predicated on fundamental revisions or reforms in the way
the existing system operated. This agreement represented
the first major policy for the evolving program.

We decided that if OEO was going to spend any substantial amounts of money on health, it would have
to be directed to changing the organizational framework through which health services were being deliv-
ered to poor people. (Schorr, 1975)

According to the interpretation of the staff, the hospital was the cornerstone of the system around which other components were linked. Any attempt at reform, therefore, ultimately would have to respond to that reality. One of the
central figures in the health program, Daniel Zwick, recalled
that:

The importance of the hospital was clear from the
beginning. Anybody who knew the business, and Lee
[Schorr] knows the business and Joe [English, Assistant Director of OEO for Health Affairs] knows
the business and Julie Richmond certainly knows
the business, would recognize the importance of the
hospital.... [We realized] that most of the medical
care that was being provided was in institutional
settings, and you had to change the hospital.
(Zwick, 1975)

Medical education was also crucial to the staff's assessment of the nature of the problem and the design for
change. Therefore, the reform agenda must also impact
schools and teaching hospitals in order to sensitize and
train health professionals to be responsive to the needs of
the poor.

A formal health services program was authorized by mid-
1965. The staff immediately developed a strategy for pursuing the broad-scale reform, grounded on a realistic assessment of the limited resources at their disposal, the professional resistance which might be anticipated, and the importance of professional visibility and legitimation.

The initial thinking emphasized the importance of providing maximum support for a small number of health centers,

in order to demonstrate most effectively the new model of
care. Accordingly, the limited resources of the program for
FY's 1965 and 1966 (a total of 9.8 million dollars) were focused on eight demonstration projects.

The health staff also realized the importance of minimizing the professional and public resistance which might be
anticipated because of perceived competition. They determined, however, that this would not be a major problem because the projects would be located in underserved areas
where few private health professionals were practicing.

The keystone of the strategy, therefore, was to initiate projects in settings where the concentration of resources
would encounter the least opposition. Mr. Zwick summarized
this thinking:

> The strategy that was being developed..., was to
> start outside that vested institution [the hospi-
> tal] . If you started within the structured
> institution you had so many things working against
> you that your chances of movement were less. So
> let's start out here with this free-standing neigh-
> borhood health center, and develop de novo without
> all of those vested interests. (Zwick, 1975)

However, the OEO health staff was also aware of the
need to establish as quickly as possible a degree of professional legitimation and recognition for the program. Such
a need assumed some association with established health institutions, particularly medical schools and teaching hospitals. This factor, for example, was key to the decision to
fund the first project through the Tufts University College
of Medicine. The Director of the agency, Mr. Shriver, recalled that he

> Was delighted that a major university and medical
> school had come forth and shown the initiative and
> let's just say the courage to propose [the project].
> That was valuable. Very valuable. (Shriver, 1976)

University sponsorship was particularly important as a
foil against the professional and public opposition which
was anticipated. Mr. Shriver stressed this point in describing his response to an application from the University of
Southern California for an NHC project in Watts.

> Well, first of all, Southern California Medical School
> was looked upon as a very good and conservative medi-
> cal school. And the Dean there was a man named

Egeberg, and he was looked upon as a very conservative Dean--I am talking about politically conservative as well as, let's say, medically conservative.
And when he said it was "Okay," my god, that was
fantastic! That was fantastic ammunition. That
was a terrific defense against an attack that
would have blown the whole thing out of the water.
Oh, there is no question about that! (Emphasis
added.) (Shriver, 1976)

The project officials at the local level were also
aware of the importance of this factor in the early strategy
of the agency. Drs. Count Gibson and Jack Geiger, the co-
directors of the Tufts Columbia Point Project, both stressed
this point in recounting the decision by OEO to fund the
first NHC project.

A key factor in overcoming Shriver's anxiety, and in
Kravitz's enthusiasm [for the Tufts project] was
that there was a major, quality medical school that
they were giving this to. I don't think that it
would have gotten started in any other way. (Geiger,
1974)

The strategy of seeking professional legitimation
through an association with established and respected hospitals and medical schools also promised to resolve other problems for the new NHC program. For example, any long-range
reform attempt assumed that the initial NHC projects would
be considered as permanent institutions, with adequate facilities and staff. The initial negotiations around the Tufts
project, according to Dr. Geiger, stressed this point.

I said,... "This is not going to be some crash program that ends up with trailers in a cotton field.
This is a university." (Geiger, 1974)

The cornerstone of this strategy rested on the assumption that gifted and innovative individuals could be located
within local health care institutions. These individuals,
functioning as local "change agents," would hold similar
views about the need to reform medical care. When provided
with adequate federal resources through the NHC program, it
was argued, the local change agent (described as a "leading-
edge, creative person") (Pugliese, 1975) could effectively
alter the philosophy and goals of the institution.

In implementing this strategy, one of the principal
criteria for evaluating the change agent was the degree to
which he/she reflected the goals and commitment of the NHC

program. Ideally, as one official recalled, the individual
would be "familiar with the notion of community health and
[have] a comprehensive orientation." These concepts of community health and comprehensive care were relatively new to
the field of medical care at the time and some members of
the health staff anticipated that "the national reservoir of
people who were au courant" would be limited. (Pugliese,
1975) At bottom, the change agent had to be cosmopolitan in
outlook, and therefore more attuned to issues at the national level. The linkage which might be established through an
NHC project was essential for both the change agent and the
health reformers. Mr. Zwick described this strategy in the
following fashion:

> My model of social reform is that change agents
> develop out in the society. Then they come to
> Washington for help and we reinforce them. And
> they're more likely to get reinforcement from a
> national program, in terms of social change, than
> they are among their fellow faculty members. But
> the fact that they get reinforced, if you're
> lucky, improves their power situation within that
> medical school and within that hospital. (Zwick,
> 1975)

In their search for "innovative" and "creative" change
agents, the OEO officials assumed that, among health care
institutions, the medical schools and teaching hospitals
would be the principal sources for such talent. Dr. Kravitz
spelled out the rationale for this initial reliance on academic physicians.

> The kind of people who were doing the... advanced
> thinking about progressive delivery of health
> care were... in universities. Those were the
> people we were relying on for consultation and
> guidance... I mean doctors in [private] practice
> don't write proposals. Health departments may
> do it, but you don't get very decent proposals
> out of them... Intellectuals write proposals.
> (Kravitz, 1975)

The notion of the university as the source of creative
experimentation was obviously widely held by the public,
and was further reinforced by the prior experiences of many
key officials in the agency, several of whom had previously
held academic appointments. This was apparent in the description by the former director of the NHC program, Dr.
John Frankel, of a dilemma which developed over the review
of a particular proposal which came to OEO directly from a

community group with no established medical institutional
sponsorship.

> Ruth Hanft and I struggled with [the application] for
> days. We kept saying, "You mean that there is no
> great medical university behind them? How can we do
> this?" But finally, we took the bit in our teeth, and
> said quite literally, "Goddamit, let's fund this
> one! It sounds good!" We had our prejudices that
> were based on everything that was in our background.
> We were quite naturally a lot more comfortable with
> a medical school or a great teaching hospital.
> (Emphasis added.) (Frankel, 1975)

The relative status of academic physicians (and thus,
of projects sponsored by medical schools and teaching hospitals) was also apparent in the early publicity accorded to
the first NHC demonstration programs. The Tufts University-
sponsored Columbia Point Project was lionized in the press
and perceived by the professional community as the embodi-
ment of the concept. For example, a conference of leaders
in the field of medical care was convened in the Spring of
1966 in New York to consider the broad issue of "health care
for the poor," and the grant to Tufts was a major focus of
discussion.[5] The director of a similar NHC grant, also a-
warded in the Summer of 1965, to the Denver Health Department, was not invited to the meeting. In retrospect, this
director, Dr. Samuel Johnson, stressed the importance of
university sponsorship as a factor in public and professional acceptance.

> I suspect that Gibson and Geiger got more calls
> [for consultation] than I did because they were
> a little bit more legitimate than I was. They
> were professors and on the faculty at a medical
> center. I was just some jerk. For one thing,
> I was west of the Mississippi, and I was running
> the Health Department. (Johnson, 1976)

The health officials in OEO clearly recognized the importance of local institutional support for the change agent.
At the same time, this was not absolutely critical and, as
one key official recalled, the OEO staff accepted the fact
that many of the change agents were relatively low in the
"pecking order" of the sponsoring institution.

> I couldn't, for the life of me, tell you what Jack
> [Geiger's] position was within the Tufts super-
> structure, for example. What was the first guy at
> Watts? Bob Tranquada. I don't know what his

position was either. The guy at St. Luke's in New
York, Paul Torrens, it seems to me, was kind of low
in the pecking order. (Pugliese, 1975)

The nature and purpose of the NHC projects presupposed
that certain administrative units within health institutions
would be more interested and supportive of the program. In
medical schools, this usually meant departments of preventive, community, and family medicine. In some instances,
NHC grants were made with the implicit understanding that
such a project would permit a designated change agent to
build up a new department. More significant for the outcome
of the strategy of institutional reform was the obvious fact
that these departments were "relatively marginal" to the
locus of power within medical schools. (Geiger, 1974)

In summary, the strategy for reforming the key health
institutions was predicated on perceived sources and levels
of opposition, as well as available resources. The OEO
health officials courted the interests of these institutions
in order to establish the legitimacy of the NHC program.
This strategy assumed that change agents could be identified
within local health institutions who would reflect the values of the national program. These individuals, usually
based in medical schools and teaching hospitals, would compete for the NHC grants and, if successful, could use the
federal resources to enhance their positions within local institutional hierarchies. In turn, the change agents would
have a greater opportunity to reorient the philosophy and
goals of the sponsoring institutions toward those espoused
by the health reformers.

Operationalizing the Problem

National Level. The definition of a social problem cus-
tomarily is followed by the process of identifying and struc-
turing a solution. According to Morse, the nature of the
organization charged with the solution is critical.

A problem is operationalized by being made the
responsibility of some new or existing organizational structure of an appropriate type [with]
flexible access to needed inputs. These conditions
having been met, the organization is to some extent
free from the bonds and constraints implicit in the
institutional environment in which it works...
Since, by definition, the solution requires institutional change, with standards and limits that are
always somewhat vague, this process of setting the
organization free to act creatively and "deviantly,"

even within limits, is crucial.   (Morse, 1969)

The flexible structure of OEO in its early phase permitted the conceptualization of the reform strategy. The staff stressed the importance of flexibility, and program operations were based on professional and personal loyalties rather than bureaucratic regulations. The selection of grant applications by the OEO staff was essentially a process of "betting on individuals in specific situations rather than on judging formal proposals." During 1965-66, Ms. Schorr typified the application review procedure as

> Getting to know the applicants, knowing the
> community they were working in, knowing the
> circumstances in which they were trying to
> start a program, and making judgments based on
> that. (Schorr, 1975)

This general tone pervaded the administrative style of the agency, and was buttressed by the example of the Director. Mr. Shriver, according to Dr. Richmond, was an "anti-bureaucrat" whose "willingness to be flexible was a great asset."

> He [Shriver] thought nothing of violating the tables
> of organization and dipping down into the bowels of
> the organization if there was someone there he
> thought that had some expertise that he wanted to
> tap. (Richmond, 1975)

The health staff consciously attempted to maintain this flexibility during 1965-66 while simultaneously attracting the interest and support of professionals in related fields. In 1965, for example, they considered the possibility of organizing a formal review board of experts from outside the agency. Dr. Richmond opposed the suggestion, arguing, according to Ms. Schorr, that "you will have to keep persuading [other] people of things that you know make sense... but may not make sense [to them]." Ms. Schorr supported this opinion, thereby maintaining a large degree of freedom from professional constraints. In retrospect, she noted the significance of that decision:

> One of the reasons we were able to pursue our ob-
> jectives as efficiently and effectively as we did
> was that we were not bogged down with satisfying
> a lot of other people's agendas. (Schorr, 1975)

Program Level. Morse contends that the degree to which a problem can be resolved is dependent on the selection of organizations at the local level to execute the goals. "The function of assigning responsiblity and granting access to resources is of special importance." He further argues that only limited effect can be achieved by assigning this respon- sibility to "existing structures" because "institutionalized biases associated with the old definition [of the problem] lead to the application of unsuitable standards." (Morse, 1969, 301-316)

The OEO reform strategy was predicated on a joint spon- sorship arrangement with existing health institutions. This choice developed from the limited resources of the program and the need to achieve professional legitimation and public acceptance. However, it was anticipated that the existing institutional biases might be neutralized through the change agent. OEO officials further reasoned that the local health institutions, particularly hospitals and medical schools, would be responsive to pressure for change because they were facing problems of their own.

Local health institutions were willing to compete for the NHC grants because the OEO program appeared to provide the opportunity to solve certain of their own needs. Teach- ing institutions, for example, viewed the NHC as a means to expand student clinical experiences. Medical schools and hospitals were also aware of the opportunity to establish a progressive and relevant posture at a time when community- oriented medicine was becoming a popular theme. Moreover, these institutions were not unmindful of the financial advan- tages which might accrue as a result of NHC sponsorship, par- ticularly in light of the decreasing support for research from other federal agencies.

The opportunity to expand the clinical teaching expe- riences for medical students was a critical factor in the decision by teaching institutions to participate in the NHC program. Ruth Hanft, one of the principal staff members dur- ing the early period, underscored this rationale in assessing the initial demonstration projects.

> No medical school is going to enter into an arrange-
> ment like that without being able to circulate medi-
> cal students or house officers through [the NHC].
> (Hanft, 1975)

Other members of the OEO staff similarly stressed the point that this was a major factor in attracting the interest of administrators of teaching institutions. For example, one key staff member recounted that the interest of the admin- istrator of a major teaching hospital, by his own admission, was based on the opportunity to obtain new "teaching material." (Pugliese, 1974)

The importance of this factor was apparent after the NHC's became operational. At Tufts, as with other projects, the degree of cooperation between the various units of the medical school and the NHC project was highest among those departments which were interested "in putting students in the centers." (Geiger, 1974) In a similar vein, the Health Department-sponsored NHC in Denver was able to attract the interest and cooperation of the city teaching hospital staff only after the latter began to lose a significant number of patients from the teaching clinics to the NHC. (Johnson, 1976)

The interest of local health institutions was also related to the fact that the NHC, as a community-based medical care model directed toward the needs of the poor, would attract publicity and enhance the status of the institution within the professional community. One project director at Tufts recalled, for example, that the University Board of Trustees overcame certain anxieties regarding the application because the

> ...grant provided a sense of mission. We scooped Harvard in this regard and so I think partly the opportunities they saw for Tufts to forge a new career were persuasive. (Gibson, 1974)

The perceived significance of NHC sponsorship for institutional status, however, varied among medical schools and teaching hospitals. According to one health official in OEO, the more established institutions were often less interested, and this stemmed from the relatively marginal position of OEO as a new agency within the federal bureaucracy.

> Even when Yale and Harvard were prepared to do something different, they couldn't face the fact of coming to OEO. They went to HEW, and by that time HEW had reached the stage in which HEW would reinforce them. And then there was a whole history around Hopkins which is kind of fun. One could discuss that at some length. But Hopkins ended up by hating OEO and going to HEW for support. (Zwick, 1975)

In addition, some health institutions were attracted to the NHC program as a means of responding to the increasing demand for public accountability. At that time, hospitals and medical schools were the focus of growing demands that their efforts be more responsive to public needs. "It was right after the riots," one OEO official recalled,

> And there was the pressure [on hospitals and medi-
> cal schools] that "We have to do something quick
> for the community." That was something that was
> certainly a pressure. (Pugliese, 1975)

The local health institutions were also attracted by
the fact that the NHC projects would provide substantial
financial support. One former OEO staff member pointed to
the importance of this in assessing the participation of the
University of Southern California.

> Why should USC all of a sudden become so benevolent
> toward Watts? Well, if there weren't two million
> dollars involved, do you think that they would have?
> Hell, no! (Maurer, 1975)

The opportunities for financial support to the sponsoring institution extended beyond the conventional "overhead"
costs and included certain types of equipment as well as
faculty salaries. OEO was willing to provide some salary
support for teaching programs, particularly in areas such as
community or family medicine, reasoning that such an effort
would have a direct impact on the service project and the
sponsoring institution. Furthermore, a certain degree of
budget flexibility for the local project director was considered by OEO officials to be an element in the overall
change agent strategy. This view was summarized by one OEO
official, in assessing the philosophy of the head of the
development division of the NHC program.

> [He] always over-funded. [He] had the theory that
> you overfunded because it gains credibility [for
> the project director], especially with the medical
> community. (Hatch, 1976)

In sum, the flexible structure of OEO, reflected in the
health office, provided the latitude to conceptualize in a
new fashion a solution to the problem of health services for
the poor. Despite the existence of traditional biases in
the existing local health institutions, the OEO officials
determined to pursue the reform strategy through those organizations, reasoning that limited resources and the need
for professional legitimacy prohibited other alternatives.
In addition, they felt that the change agent, reflecting
their own views, could balance the traditional biases. A
critical point in this logic was the assumption that the perceived problems of local institutions would make them recep-
tive to the proposed reforms. The local institutions did

compete for NHC grants because sponsorship seemed to provide, in the short run, a mechanism for resolving existing dilemmas.

Epilogue: Reform Strategy in a Shifting Milieu

The NHC program was enlarged significantly in 1967, following the passage of legislation which provided more precise authorization and earmarked approximately 50 million dollars for new projects. This expansion coincided with a reorganization within OEO which expanded the role and status of the NHC program. Additional staff were added and greater attention was focused on operational and managerial procedures, activities directed toward institutional maintenance types of functions.

The shift in emphasis away from specific goal functions ("comprehensive care", "community based") was evidenced by the increasing orientation of the staff to issues beyond the customary purview of health services innovations. For example, one key official reasoned that the expanded publicity, both in the general public and the Congress, required greater attention to "the politics of it." The increased size of the program meant that "the enemies that you make become a lot more important and you need a lot more friends." (Schorr, 1975) Consequently, the administration of the program was more sensitive to the possibility of locating NHC projects in the districts of key legislators. Moreover, greater efforts were made to respond to the interests and opposition of local officials.

The process of growth, bureaucratization, and shift in institutional function obviously affected the degree of innovation that was possible. Ms. Schorr, who witnessed this change, summarized it in the following way:

> I think there is also a big question of whether it is possible to maintain the kind of spirit and atmosphere... when you get bigger, because the kinds of personal relationships... and a lot of personal trust... that were really the underpinning no longer worked when you have that many people involved....
> And when you begin to codify some of these decisions that were made very casually and very informally, you get a different atmosphere. I think it is harder for the kinds of people who were interested and very innovative and very creative, to work in that atmosphere. (Emphasis added.) (Schorr, 1975)

Coincident with these developments (1967-68), evidence began to surface from the program level which forced OEO health officials to question the initial reform strategy. The sponsoring institutions, and medical schools in particular, were not responding in a way which had been anticipated. This judgment was grounded on the continuing problem of negotiating a realistic overhead charge, the disagreement as to appropriate use of salaried staff, and evidence of the lack of interest on the part of the administrations of the sponsoring institutions. Any interest or enthusiasm which was present initially had clearly dissipated, because, as one official judged, the basic "commitment" was not present to begin with.

> I am hard-pressed to think of a university medical
> center that handled itself in a mode of real commit-
> ment to the program, rather than being dragged in,
> or seduced in, or whatever the mechanism was.
> (Pugliese, 1975)

This realization was reflected in the decrease of new grants to medical school sponsors. Thirty-seven percent of all new grants made during 1965-66 went to medical schools. In the following year, this decreased to 18 percent, and continued to fall to 11 percent in 1968. This change was accompanied by a less precipitate but steady decline in new projects awarded to hospitals (excepting 1969). Corresponding to these two changes was an increase in the percentage of new project grants awarded to new health corporations, such as incorporated neighborhood councils. Table 1, adapted from data developed by Zwick (1972), outlines these changes.

Table 1. Types of neighborhood health center-sponsoring institutions at the time of initial grant award, 1965-71.

INSTITUTION	YEAR					
	1965-66	1967	1968	1969	1970	1971
	%	%	%	%	%	%
New health corpora- tion	-	24	33	33	52	59
Hospital	50	21	22	67	9	10
Medical school	37	18	11	-	18	7
Others	13	35	33	-	22	24

Although these changes were partially in response to the increasing pressure for citizen participation and control, they nonetheless represented a realization that the reform strategy, to the degree initially anticipated, was no longer viable. In subsequent years, new project awards were made to hospitals and medical schools. However, these do not represent a revival of the reform strategy, but rather a response to the policy changes adopted by the Nixon administration.

The denouement of the reform goal was clearly apparent by 1969, although the health staff continued to use the language for rhetorical and inspirational purposes. It was a direct result of new policies imposed by the Nixon administration which found broad popular support in a radically altered social and political milieu. This policy effectively shifted the activities of the NHC program toward institutional maintenance functions. Although the funding for the OEO program doubled in 1969 and increased thereafter, these policies eliminated any remaining vestiges of organizational orientation toward specific goal functions.

The goal of the new policy was to permit the expansion of the NHC program, but within a framework consistent with the views of the new administration. The initial stage was to move the authority for the program to an appropriate agency within the more established and conservative D/HEW. Shortly after taking office in 1969, the new administration organized a planning task force for this purpose; the actual transfer occurred during 1971-72 (Hanft, 1975):

The goals of this new policy were more immediately made manifest in a series of new regulations. These guidelines were justified on the grounds of enhancing the efficiency and management of the program. At the same time, whether by accident or design, they also expanded the paperwork enormously and delayed the operational and administrative processes (Hatch, 1976). In response, the staff was forced to spend increasing amounts of time and energy to comply in order to keep the existing NHC projects functioning. As a result, they became further preoccupied with activities directed toward institutional maintenance functions.

Conclusion

The principal concern of the health staff within OEO during the initial phase was to establish a commitment by that agency to a new form of health services delivery for the poor. This necessitated the development and demonstration of a viable and effective model. The health staff reasoned that the existing health care system was a part of the problem and devised a reform agenda as an integral part of their goals. Toward this end, the staff effectively defined the problem and established a strategy for the operationalization of change.

The decision to operationalize the change under the aegis of existing institutions was predicated on the limited resources of the program and the need for rapid professional legitimation. These and other reasons, to their mind, preempted any serious consideration of an alternative model of social change, viz., the formation of new institutions free from existing biases.

The strategy for the reform agenda focused on a local surrogate who would hold similar views and use the NHC program and resources as leverage for change within the sponsoring institution. The seeming naivete of this expectation must be balanced by the knowledge that the local sponsoring institution knowingly entered into a NHC contract which made explicit many elements of the reform agenda.

The sponsoring institutions were attracted by the opportunity to use the NHC project to resolve specific problems of their own. As resolution occurred, or the liabilities of sponsorship increased, local institutions became less committed to the faithful execution of the contract and withdrew from active participation. Elsewhere, we have argued that much of the conflict which later surfaced between OEO and the sponsoring institutions was directly related to basic differences in goal orientation (May, et al., forthcoming).

In devising and executing their agenda, the health reformers made certain assumptions about the supporting social and political milieu. Consequently, their initial plan of action focused primarily on the "demonstration" of the model and was only marginally involved with documentation and evaluation. As Morse and others have stressed, this freedom from conventional constraints, even customary data constraints, is absolutely essential for the definition of an innovation (Morse, 1969). Subsequent critiques which point to the inadequacy of the uniform data reporting and management information systems during the initial period are therefore inappropriate because they fail to grasp this essential element of the process of social change.

The effective demonstration of the model led to a period of significant expansion, which in turn tended to orient the activities of the program toward system maintenance functions. The conventional process of bureaucratization, however, was later exaggerated when a new administration sought to limit the program by applying extensive and rigorous guidelines. Freedom of action, therefore, became a casualty of this structure and, while actual program expansion proceeded, the emphasis on system maintenance functions, for purposes of protection, effectively excluded any substantive reform.

The question of the overall success/failure of the NHC program is beyond the purview of this paper. Such a judgment would require the identification of discrete goals (the quality and extent of services provided, the degree of institutional change effected, the extent of "demonstration" of the model, etc.) and the organization of appropriate data. The existing evaluations, as Hollister and Kramer (1974) forcefully argued earlier, tend to focus on relatively minor issues where data abounds, and ignore other goals of the program which are more complex and less amenable to quantitative analysis, such as training and education, or citizen participation.

Our purpose has been to define the strategy of the program and analyze it within the context of institutional change. In turn, we propose that this framework will permit a more exact analysis of the degree of change within those health institutions as a result of NHC project sponsorship. Such an effort will allow a more precise judgment of the outcome of the reform agenda.

Notes

1. Nine of the respondents (four OEO officials and five project directors) who were particularly important to the NHC program and to the study were re-interviewed, bringing the total number of interviews to 88.

2. The specific positions which the respondents held are as follows:
    Federal officials - 44
        OEO staff - 37
        Congressional staff - 2
        D/HEW officials - 3
        Federal contractors - 2

    Program officials - 35
        Project directors - 24
        Project administrators - 7
        Community board leaders - 4

Between January, 1974, and December, 1977, a total of 150 hours of interviews were conducted, recorded, and transcribed, with the average interview lasting one hour and forty minutes.

The initial contact letter to each respondent described the project (an "Oral History of the Neighborhood Health Center Movement"), cited the support of various organizations, and detailed the steps which had been arranged to protect the confidence of the respondents. The introductory letter was followed by a telephone call which included additional information and scheduled the date of the interview.

A standard set of data was collected on each respondent which included the following: information on the respondent drawn from previous interviews, published materials, and information from earlier studies; the respondent's curriculum vitae and copies of any professional writings; correspondence and notes from telephone conversations; extensive field notes on each respondent developed by the interviewers. This information, plus the transcriptions of the interviews, provided the basis for this paper.

A copy of the interview is in the possession of the respondents. The future use of the materials will be determined by each respondent and the National Association of Community Health Centers, Inc. The co-investigators anticipate that at the conclusion of the project a copy of most interviews will be deposited in an appropriate archive.

3. There were two exceptions to the sampling. The investigators completed interviews with all persons who had served as project directors in three specific centers. Secondly, in one center, interviews were completed with several key community board leaders.

A total of 82 potential respondents were contacted by mail and telephone, and three declined to participate in the study. A more detailed analysis of the reasons for this degree of cooperation is included in Jude Thomas May and Peter K. New, "101% Response Rate: Reflections on Over-Cooperation in an Interview-Based Study of Health Policy." Paper presented at the meetings of the Society for Applied Anthropology, April, 1977, Dan Diego.

4. Dr. Gibson described the incident as he learned of it from a participant at the meeting, Dr. Alonzo Yerby. Interview, Dr. Gibson.

5. "1966 Health Conference of the New York Academy of Medicine," held in New York, April 21-22, 1966. Several of the papers were subsequently published in the Bulletin of the New York Academy of Medicine, 42, 12 (December, 1966), including Lisbeth Bamberger (Schorr), "Health Care and Poverty," pp. 1140-49, which precisely outlines the early goals and spirit of the program.

References

Frankel, John. Interview, January 23, 1975.

Geiger, H. Jack. Interview, June 26, 1974.

Gibson, Count D. Interview, March 4, 1974.

Hanft, Ruth. Interview, June 16, 1975.

Hatch, Lucia. Interview, June 16, 1976.

Hollister, Robert M. "Neighborhood Health Centers as Demonstrations." Chapter in Robert M. Hollister, Bernard M. Kramer, and Seymour S. Bellin, eds. Neighborhood Health Centers. Lexington, Mass.: Lexington Books, 1974.

Johnson, Samuel. Interview, June 2, 1976.

Kravitz, Sanford. Interview, October 9, 1975.

Maurer, Sidney. Interview, July 30, 1975.

May, J. T., Peter K. New, L.R. Judd, and E.J. Anderson. The Neighborhood Health Center Program, Its Growth and Problems: An Introduction. Washington: National Association of Community Health Centers, Inc., 1976.

May, Jude Thomas and Peter K. New. "101% Response Rate: Reflections on Over-Cooperation in an Interview-Based Study of Health Policy." Paper presented at the meetings of the Society for Applied Anthropology, April, 1977, San Diego.

May, Jude Thomas, Mary Durham, and Peter K. New, "Structural Conflicts in the Neighborhood Health Center Program: The National and Local Perspectives." Forthcoming, Journal of Health Politics, Policy and Law.

Morse, Chandler. "Becoming Versus Being Modern: An Essay on Institutional Change and Economic Development." Chapter in C. Morse, et al., <u>Modernization by Design: Social Change in the Twentieth Century</u>. Ithaca: Cornell University Press, 1969.

New York Academy of Medicine. <u>Bulletin of the New York Academy of Medicine</u>, 42, 12 (December, 1966): 1140-1149.

Pugliese, Donald. Interview, April 11, 1975.

Richmond, Julius. Interview, November 4, 1975.

Schorr, Lee B. Interview, October 16, 1975.

Schorr, Lisbeth B. and Joseph T. English. "Background, Context and Significant Issues in Neighborhood Health Center Programs." <u>Milbank Memorial Fund Quarterly</u>, 66, 3, part 1 (July, 1968): 289-296.

Shriver, Sargent. Interview, June 18, 1976.

Zwick, Daniel I. Interview, May 13, 1975.

Zwick, Daniel I. "Some Accomplishments and Findings of Neighborhood Health Centers." <u>Milbank Memorial Fund Quarterly</u>, 50, 4, Part 1 (October, 1972): 387-420.

Part 2

Sociocultural and Psychobiological Dynamics

_____ *Anne Mooney, Thomas J. Nagy*

Introduction: Part 2

The first part of this volume emphasized the social system level of analysis from the perspectives of the disciplines of sociology, demography, economics, and politics. At this level of analysis, two types of problems can be studied: (1) differences in health levels among populations living under different social systems, and (2) the health effects of changes in a given social system. Prominent among the latter changes are trends and fluctuations in the socioeconomic characteristics of the social system.

In introducing Part 1, Ratcliffe described an emergent paradigm that attributes changes in mortality fundamentally to socioeconomic aspects of economic development. High-priority research topics in this field include specification of: (1) the aspects of economic development that are beneficial, or harmful, to health; (2) the sorts of persons or communities at particularly high risk, given certain economic changes; (3) the mechanisms that translate economic changes into pathology, and interventions most likely to minimize such consequences; and (4) a conceptualization of the entire process from economic change to health outcome that is both accurate and comprehensible to the public and to policy makers.

In order to account for variations in characteristics—including social status and health status—among people living in the same social system, analyses are required using concepts that relate individual personalities and social positions to the social system. The sociocultural view presented in **Part 2 of the volume focuses on human behavior as explicated in the disciplines of anthropology, social psychology,** psychiatry, and psychology. The elements of culture—symbols, values, beliefs, and social structure—come to the fore; phenomena are treated as they are experienced at the individual level.

A bridge from the social system level of analysis in
Part 1 to the sociocultural materials in Part 2 is provided by
Gonzalez in a wide-ranging review of the contributions of anthropological research to health, covering the areas of cultural definitions of health and illness, social organization
in health and illness, and environmental effects on health.
She treats topics as diverse as the medical value of indigenous beliefs; challenges to the assumption that illness is
simply the reflection of unusual physical conditions; the role
of the social network and mutual aid societies in the reco- ⁄
very of health; and the effects on health of factors external
to individuals and their societies.

The papers by Schofield and Greenley develop two important
issues with respect to health differentials in modern socie-
ties--psychosocial factors in susceptibility to illness and
factors related to differences in utilization of health care
services. Notwithstanding the influence of macro-socioecono-
mic factors on health, substantial numbers of people remain
healthy even under adverse conditions. Schofield suggests
that differences in patterns of perceiving events and in
coping styles can explain the difference in outcomes among
persons facing the same pattern of stress. If the determinants of these particular psychological differences can be
understood, then persons might be taught to adapt in a more
healthy fashion to stress which cannot be avoided. Furthermore, as persons at high risk for given illnesses are more
accurately identified, they might be sought out and taught to
alter their behaviors in ways designed to minimize morbidity
and mortality. The power of social networks and self-help
groups to assist in the treatment of disease, as noted by
Gonzalez, might be mobilized to prevent disease by assisting
highly susceptible persons to alter self-destructive behaviors.

Schofield explains the influence of psychosocial factors
on susceptibility to physical illness. He concentrates on
life situations that lower resistence and increase susceptibility because they are perceived in a way that creates tension. Noting that the relationship between situational stress
and illness shows a consistent but low association, Schofield
offers a research agenda including detailed studies of the
interaction between situational crises and life style, the
study of resistent persons as well as susceptibles, and large-
scale prospective studies.

Much of the social-science research in health has been
directed toward understanding the social organization of
health care. Gonzalez examines the topic both with respect
to patient support by family and community and to social
organization of medical practitioners. Greenley has provided

a detailed, critical review of the literature of one aspect of medical care, namely, utilization of services. His review of "socio-cultural and psychological aspects of utilization of health services" begins by noting that the topic was first investigated to understand problems of unequal distribution of health services. More recently, interest has turned to overutilization, a most difficult topic for investigation since perceptions of a proper level of care are the products of social and cultural factors rather than medical-scientific outcomes.

Utilization is a multidimensional phenomenon whose various aspects are relatively uncorrelated with one another. Furthermore, no overall theory of utilization exists. While sociodemographic factors, morbidity, income, ethnicity, beliefs, and attitudes, propensity to adopt the sick role, as well as alienation, fatalism, and psychological distress all play a role in utilization, Greenley concludes that substantial progress has been achieved in understanding utilization and points to strategies for building on the previous studies.

An historical analysis of social science contributions to medical care and medical education, including suggestions for enhancing utilization of social science in medicine, are provided by Reiser. The medical curriculum still remains largely in the physical and biological science framework proposed by Flexner. While pioneers like Cabot recognized the centrality of understanding social conditions in treating patients, concern for this realm fell entirely to the social service personnel which he organized. The social service idea spread, but "by allowing physicians to delegate responsibility for learning about the social factors, it seems to have reduced their own need to comprehensively master the knowledge that the social sciences could contribute."

Reiser asserts that the greatest success of the social sciences in medicine has been to delineate the cultural and social factors influencing sickness and calls for more work in assessing the outcome of medical interventions in terms of social and cultural variables, as well as the operational use of social science in direct clinical care. To the extent that these efforts are successfully pursued, the policy relevance of social science at the sociocultural level will be much enhanced.

4. Cultural and Environmental Factors in the Definition and Understanding of Health

Serious anthropological interest in the relationship between culture and health status began in the 1940's. John Bennett, Margaret Mead, and a few others did work in the general area that I will here call "beliefs and practices". Most of this work was descriptive, and one of its main results was to persuade physicians and other health personnel that non-Western peoples possessed (and were possessed by) indigenous medical systems. The "fallacy of the empty vessels," as Polgar put it (1962), had previously held that tribal and peasant peoples had no medical knowledge whatever, and that all that was needed in order to improve their health was instruction in modern (i.e., Western) beliefs and practices.

Even after this attitude was abandoned, it was frequently assumed that the existing indigenous beliefs and practices were false and that they must be changed or eliminated so that others might be introduced and adopted. Herbal and other indigenous remedies were thought to be useless, and modern remedies were urged upon peoples all over the world.

Many practices were thought to be based upon superstition and/or ignorance of anatomy and physiology. A striking example of our ethnocentrism in this regard is the notion that childbirth is best accomplished in a horizontal, reclining position, a largely Western practice which some suggest is beneficial for no one except, perhaps, the attending physician. Much attention was paid to "improving" diets simply because they were very different from what we were used to. Although it is true that dietary deficiency diseases have been prevalent in some parts of the world, we now know that it is primarily poverty rather than ignorance which results in a poorly nourished population. Most indigenous dietary regimes are probably highly satisfactory, even when they include foods and culinary practices of which our culture might disapprove, such as cannibalism or vegetarianism.

One of the most important contributions of anthropologists to the health field in recent years has been the suggestion that many indigenous beliefs and practices may be as good or better than our own. These are more and more being studied to determine their intrinsic value, and in some cases are now being urged upon the American public. Recent interest in dietary fiber is an example. The well known hot/cold classification of foods and bodily conditions in Latin American countries, a legacy of Hippocrates, has long been thought to be purely magical. However, recently it has been suggested that some of the related behavior patterns may contribute to maintenance of electrolyte balance, and perhaps should be examined in greater detail by epidemiologists and medical anthropologists (McCullough, 1973). Of course, even "magical" rites may have powerful curing potential due to the psychological well-being they produce.

On the other hand, a careful examination of our own culture shows that we also have beliefs and practices which defy scientific explanation, but which most of us would insist are at least partially efficacious. Ironically, perhaps, the attention of applied social scientists was first directed to non-Western medical systems so that public health personnel might work more efficiently in foreign lands or among American Indians. However, increased knowledge of the rest of the world has led us to view our own ways in a new light. Even the educated middle class "middle American" uses home remedies, engages in some magical and ritual practices, but ultimately turns to culturally approved and "anointed" medical specialists when the condition worsens or persists. This is no different from what anthropologists have found in societies throughout the world.

Another result of studies at home has been the recognition and documentation of the variations in beliefs and practices which exist in our own society, results of different ethnic backgrounds and levels of formal education. "Folk culture" is just as much a part of our own system as it is in parts of Mexico, Sri Lanka, or Nigeria.

Following the "beliefs and practices" stage, anthropologists began to realize that health itself and the ways in which people define disease and illness are themselves culturally determined. Symptoms of ill health vary tremendously in terms of what they mean functionally to the individuals who have them. For example, in some societies, among certain classes of people, diarrhea may be chronic, "normal", and therefore no cause for alarm. Vertigo, fainting, and hallucinations may be considered symptoms of divine favor, and persons with such conditions may be urged to join priesthoods or become shamans. Sometimes they are themselves worshipped or considered holy. Finally, taking an example from an earlier period in our own history, skin eruptions may be thought to be the result of masturbation and/or poor hygiene, and in any case "natural" in adolescence.

What Fabrega (1975) has called "bio-medicine", a product of Western civilization, concerns itself with the physiological conditions ("disease") underlying the culturally defined symptoms ("illness"). It has generally been accepted that human physiology is everywhere the same (but I shall elaborate on that a little later), and thus, a physician well trained in bio-medicine should be able to diagnose and treat symptoms in any population. But cure turns out to vary independently of biomedical prescriptions. The behavioral and social components of disease (which constitute the "illness") are not so well handled, largely because these are not universal and because a special knowledge of each culture is necessary for full understanding. For this the physician needs professional social scientific guidance or training.

Close participant observation of how the members of the society treat the person manifesting certain symptoms can tell us much about whether the condition is recognized as an illness at all, and whether it is regarded as being serious or mild. (See Ohnuki-Tierney, 1978, for an illuminating discussion.) In our society, for example, most educated persons pay relatively little attention to what we call "colds." The sick person often does little or nothing for treatment, and only rarely seeks professional medical help. Among the Jicaque of Honduras, on the other hand, a cold is a most serious matter, and a great deal of societal attention is paid to it. The fact that few persons in our society ever die of a cold, while the Jicaque have historically succumbed in large numbers, is basic to an understanding of the different behaviors involved. While we seek merely symptomatic relief and wait it out, the Jicaque have constructed a much more elaborate system for handling both the condition and its prevention. Fear of illness led them, until very recently, to resist visits from outsiders, regardless of their purpose and affiliation. Consequently, they remained isolated for a longer period from the mainstream of Honduran national society than might otherwise have been the case.[1]

True "illness" in any culture usually implies a certain

level of disability. So long as it is possible to go about
one's usual activities with only minor behavioral changes,
one may not be considered "really" ill, although the threshold may be somewhat different for different people. Each
society has a more or less standardized set of acceptable
"sick roles" which demand recognition and a certain amount of
sympathy, if not serious concern. In our own society, a
day's absence once a month for working women is tolerated.
Some chronic conditions may even, among certain social
classes, become status symbols. Gout was once thought to affect only the rich and well fed. Paleness, frailty and thin-
ness were, and to a certain extent still are, symbolic of
feminine beauty, particularly among the more affluent classes. Significantly, the lower classes seem always to have
prefered a more robust figure, perhaps because robustness is
thought to imply better health and a greater ability to work.

On the other hand, we find that certain conditions demand definition as illness, regardless of the level of pain
or degree of physical disability associated with them. Cancer, leprosy, epilepsy, and, especially, spastic and paraplegic conditions fall into this category in our society. It
is also interesting to examine what happens in our society
in regard to the use of sick leave. In most cases, this
leave cannot be accumulated, but is lost when unused after a
certain period of time. But if one does exhaust it, and especially if one goes beyond it, even though the leave is un-
paid, the person may earn a reputation for being in poor
health and, consequently, be thought a poor employment risk.
In time, such a person may adopt or be forced into a "chronically sick" role, which may help compensate for the loss of
employment through increased sympathy and, sometimes, disability payments. So far, the Office of Health, Education
and Welfare has not challenged an employer's prerogative to
reject an applicant because of chronic or frequent ill
health, even though discrimination against some of the conditions listed above (the paraplegic, for example) is frowned
upon. However, obesity, even though associated with a propensity for disease (diabetes, hypertension, e.g.) may not
be used as a basis for terminating employment.

It is also significant to note that there are certain
conditions which are ambiguously defined. Only in recent
years have alcoholism and homosexuality been classified as
diseases, and some would still disagree with such a statement. This assumes the possiblity of "cure" or reversal of
the condition, and places great weight on societal factors
in etiology. Using similar criteria, Fabrega (1975) has suggested that unemployment might be said to constitute an illness, and that we might eventually define it as such in our

society. Fabrega's argument is persuasive to the extent that society can alter individuals' behavior, sometimes to the point that individuals are incapacitated or rendered incapable of carrying out normal life roles.

Recently the senior U.S. Senator from California, Alan Cranston, has voiced the thought that aging itself might be considered a reversible condition, thus putting it and its symptoms into the category of illness, as Fabrega uses that term (Cranston, 1978). Certainly it is often true that the elderly are treated as though they were chronically ill. I foresee increasing scientific and public interest in this area in the near future.

The social sciences have had a modicum of success in demonstrating the importance of culture in defining illness and disease. However, another more important impact has resulted from research on the social organization of health and illness. This includes not only the study of patient support systems such as the family and community, but also the study of the social organization of the medical practitioners themselves. Although social scientists have long been aware that we should not treat the sick one as an isolated individual, and although this idea has been taught in schools of medicine and of nursing, I believe it is still the case that most physicians and other Western medical personnel continue to think and act as though the patient were an island. Although close relatives may be consulted if the patient is extremely weak or dying, more often they are excluded except when they are financially responsible or needed to carry out medical orders in the home. At a recent conference on problems of infantile malnutrition in developing countries, the physicians in attendance dwelled almost exclusively on the sick children and their mothers. There was an almost total absence of reference to anyone else within the society, as well as a failure to appreciate the multiplicity of roles occupied by the woman. For this group she existed only as "mother," and in the words of one participant, "cow."

This is in extreme contrast with societies such as that of the South African Bushmen, or San, among whom illness is treated communally. The entire family and often the whole band gathers about the sick one, and the medicine men perform rituals thought to benefit the whole group.

Still, our society has other ways of mobilizing, almost in spite of the formal medical system. Visits to hospitalized persons are often discouraged, and seldom prescribed. Therefore, we send flowers, cards, and gifts to sick friends

to show our moral support. Such symbols are important psychologically and probably contribute to the recovery of the
patient. They demonstrate that the sick one is valued and
an integral part of a social network.

Epidemiologists are aware of the importance of social
networks in spreading disease. Gadjusek's explanation of
the transmission of kuru in New Guinea is particularly dramatic and now quite well known (Gadjusek, 1977). However,
those physicians concerned with curing or therapy often seem
not to recognize that these same social networks may be utilized to enhance the well-being of the patient.

However, we must also examine how social status changes
when certain conditions, usually chronic or permanent ones,
become manifest. Such illnesses as leprosy, cancer, alcoholism, and multiple sclerosis will indeed alter the person's position, and, in many cases, effectively remove the
individual from all previously existing networks of which he
or she was a part. Although a great deal of progress has
been made in our understanding of these conditions and in the
importance of maintaining the social linkages, there are
still thousands of cases in which the ill one is placed in
an institution. Even without institutionalization, there is
likely to be a reduction in the number and quality of interpersonal contacts with earlier friends and with relatives.
Homosexuals, if identified, are also isolated from previously existing support systems, as are accident victims who
lose mobility through loss of sight, hearing, or limbs. In
such cases, as in many of those mentioned above, the emphasis tends to shift away from family and earlier associates
toward others in a similar condition.

Social scientists are only now beginning to examine in
detail the structure and functioning of supportive voluntary
associations. Many follow the model of Alcoholics Anonymous,
a long established and quite successful organization which
has, through the years, developed a set of rituals, symbols,
and prescriptive social relationships serving to help the
uncontrolled alcoholic and support those susceptible to re-
lapse.

A listing of such formalized mutual aid societies related to health problems would be long and would probably
surprise many health workers. Their popularity seems at
least partially attributable to the need for chronically ill
or handicapped persons to create their own networks in the
face of rejection or misunderstanding on the part of relatives and neighbors. Yet to say this is superficial in the
extreme. We need to study the symbolic, as well as the

social, mechanisms which develop among these groups. They are products of a complex society, as are many of the diseases and conditions from which they spring. We must further examine the linkages between mutual aid societies and other components of the larger sociocultural system in terms of economics and political action, as well as health.

Although we do not yet totally understand the stigma and the isolation to which persons deviating from the norm are subjected, social scientists are making headway. Yet, it will be a long time before the general public will listen to, much less accept, some of their conclusions. It is interesting that last year when Dr. Joan Ablon received funding for research on the "Little People of America," the National Science Foundation would not permit the word "dwarf" to appear in the title of her grant. I attribute this to a reluctance, even on the part of highly educated scientists, to face up to the kinds of issues to which we are addressing ourselves today. Undoubtedly, they were afraid of being criticized by the general public for carrying out work on "silly," nonessential, or sensitive subjects. This fear itself may be seen as a form of prejudice.

Studies of social organization among medical personnel are also an important research area. We now understand quite well the nature of professional hierarchies, ways in which the different practitioner classes interrelate amongst themselves, and the symbols which convey meaning and preserve the system, both internally and in the eyes of the public. Even the role of popular culture (Marcus Welby, Rex Morgan) has been explored in this connection.

We are less sure of how this social organization relates directly to the curing function itself, but there are some provocative studies comparing, for example, attitudes toward chiropractors with those toward M.D.'s. The relatively low status of psychiatrists within the M.D. hierarchy may reflect what are perceived as low rates of "cure." But then how do we explain a similarly low status for pediatricians? But space does not permit a fuller examination of these issues here.

The question of environment and its effects on health is complex. Under "environment" I include a variety of factors external to the individual and the society, including the presence of other societies of humans or non-humans. Let me give a few examples.

A poor or irregular food supply, resulting in general or specific malnutrition, may be caused by unusual aridity, changes in the migration of game animals, or competition with encroaching human neighbors. In more highly developed economies, certain components of the population may become poorly nourished through an inability to purchase food during periods of recession and increased unemployment. In some cases, these circumstances may in turn have been affected by environmental factors, for example, crop failure on a large scale.

The presence or absence of intestinal or other parasites and bacteria may itself be considered an environmental factor which may also be affected by other environmental conditions. In warm moist climates infection is more difficult to control. Population size and density, also related to the interplay between technology and environment, are further factors in the control of infectious disease.

High altitude and extremes of temperature can have profound impact on health, but the human body seems able to adapt physiologically to these conditions. It is not clear whether the adaptations reflect an inherent general biological plasticity or some genetic variation resulting from the operation of selective pressures in certain populations.

Biological anthropologists have stressed that human beings are not the same all over the world. Many of the genetic differences relating to differential health status among human populations manifest themselves only in relation to variations in environment and culture. In a symposium sponsored by the AAAS last year at Denver several researchers, including Baruch Blumberg, John Eaton, Peter Bennett, and H.H. Draper gave examples of how differences in nutritional status among and within human populations may be attributable to both biological and environmental factors (Gottesman, 1977). For example, it is now well recognized that in some populations large numbers of persons are unable to digest lactose. Draper reported that among some Eskimos there may be a genetically linked sucrose intolerance. Such findings should have, but I believe have not yet had, much influence on the practicing health professions. Unfortunately, it seems to take a very long time between the original research and its translation into practice, especially in the less developed countries.

In 1956 and 1957, when I first carried out field work in Central America among black populations, I found no physician at either the village or the national level who had ever heard of sickle cell anemia. In 1975, on the other hand, I found considerable sophistication among Belizean physicians concerning this disease. In fact, a National Health

Service program for early diagnosis had been established to test the blood of all pregnant women seeking medical attention. If at this time I found a less than desirable understanding of the genetic basis of the disease, and of the possibilities for treatment and prevention, this is not surprising, considering the fact that we are still in the dark about many of these things even in the more sophisticated centers of learning. The possibility that the disease is in one way or another linked with dietary patterns has yet to be fully explored in the field, for example. Nevertheless, I think it fair to say that there has been progress, and that new knowledge does eventually filter down to local and "folk" levels. We could have a greater impact if epidemiologists, physicians, anthropologists, and others who conduct research in less developed countries would work more closely with the local medical personnel, treating them as full research partners and conducting guest lectures or classes for the local medical schools or societies. Greater attention also needs to be paid to educating the public in such countries.

Finally, I would like to speak briefly about sociobiology as a potentially useful approach in explaining certain health-related social and cultural patterns. Epidemiologists, as mentioned above, do look at kin groups and their role in caring for the sick. We know that certain social mechanisms can help reduce morbidity and mortality, increase fertility, or even assist in maintaining lower birth rates when the limits of the food supply are reached (Wynne-Edwards, 1962). The trick has always been to have <u>enough</u> but not too <u>many</u> members of the society. Either extreme leads to ultimate extinction. No doubt many societies have not achieved a satisfactory balance and have become extinct. But anthropologists today are increasingly interested in the interactions between specific social and cultural patterns, health, and the viability of the population. Van den Berghe and Barash (1977) have outlined various ways in which kinship systems and other aspects of social organization have contributed to the maintainance of an optimum population size. Even if one does not wish to invoke the concepts of "kin selection," "altruism," or "inclusive fitness" (Hamilton, 1964), it is clear that cooperative ties, reciprocity, and the protection given kin as a matter of obligation in all societies must have an important bearing upon health and, consequently, upon fitness. At least one archaeologist (Blanton, 1975) has utilized such concepts in trying to explain the dynamics of population growth in prehistoric societies.

To give some specific examples, culturally prescribed marriage at either a very early or too late an age will

present greater hazards for both mother and child and thus
contribute to a reduction in fertility. In the case of cannibalism we should contrast the dangers of spreading disease, as in kuru, with the beneficial effects of increased
protein intake. Ideologies differ: what to us seems an
abomination may be a religious rite in other times and
places.

Attitudes about breast feeding and ritual bodily mutila-
tions must also be viewed in relation to their long range impact upon the viability of the population as opposed to their
effects upon the individuals concerned. Again, even for the
individual, we must consider both biological and cultural
"risks". Clitoridectomy may be deemed indispensable for pre-
serving social status in some Ethiopian societies, even
though it presents some risk of infection.

In summary, I have tried to outline various ways in
which social science has contributed to a better understanding of the cultural and environmental factors affecting
health and disease. Within the social sciences, the domains
of health and medicine have become very popular subjects.
In anthropology, my own field, we have seen the rise of a
new professional association, the Society for Medical Anthropology; and the birth of three new journals devoted to
health subjects within the past few years.[2] In sociology,
the development of interest in health has been comparable,
and, although the methodologies used and the particular topics studied sometimes differ, all in all, sociological and
anthropological contributions reinforce and complement each
other.

Social scientists are increasingly employed in medical
settings. They are found teaching in medical and nursing
schools, working in public health clinics both at home and
abroad, and in some cases acting as consultants to particular
groups of physicians or local governments. I must caution
medical personnel, however, that a few lectures or courses
in sociology or anthropology cannot be expected to give them
more than an appreciation of the role of social, cultural,
and environmental factors in health and disease. Their own
observations, if based upon existing interpretations, understandings, and theories provided by social scientists, may
well be valid and useful in their work. But they should understand that new discoveries and theoretical groundbreaking
will continue to occur, and they should not assume that social science as yet has all the answers.

Much of what we think we know may turn out to be false,
and we must persistently delve beneath the surface of the

all too apparent "beliefs and practices" to see how these change through time and in response to environmental pressures placed upon both individuals and societies. The introduction of modern Western medical practices has occurred all over the world, though with varying acceptance rates and results. This is only one dimension of the process of acculturation, which has generated a tremendous body of literature, both descriptive and theoretical in nature.

Social scientists, especially medical anthropologists, realize that the field is still very new. We recognize that we must develop greater sophistication in the biological and medical sciences, and that we do better when we collaborate with professionals in such fields. I believe we can look forward to increasing mutual respect and closer working relations in the future. This in turn should lead to still undreamed of progress in our understanding and control of illness and disease.

Notes

1. Personal communication, Dr. Anne Chapman.

2. These are as follows:
    (1) <u>Medical Anthropology: Cross Cultural Studies in Health and Illness</u>, Redgrave Publishing Co., New York.
    (2) <u>Culture, Medicine and Psychiatry: An International Journal of Comparative Cross-Cultural Research</u>, D. Reidel, Dordecht, The Netherlands.
    (3) <u>Social Science and Medicine</u>, Pergamon Press, Oxford, England.

References

Blanton, Richard E. "The Cybernetic Analysis of Human Population Growth." Pp. 116-126 in A.C. Swedlund, ed., <u>Population Studies in Archaeology and Biological Anthropology: A Symposium</u>. Washington, D.C.: Society for American Archaeology, 1975.

Cranston, Alan. "Why Aren't We Doing More to Extend Lifespan?" Unpublished manuscript, 1978.

Fabrega, Horacio. "The Need for an Ethnomedical Science." <u>Science</u> 189 (1975): 969.

Gajdusek, Carleton. "Unconventional Viruses in the Origin and Disappearance of Kuru." <u>Science</u> 192 (1977): 943-960.

Gottesman, Irving S. "Differences in Nutritional Requirements Among and Within Human Populations: Their Significance." Symposium at 143rd Annual Meeting of the AAAS, Denver, February, 1977.

Hamilton, W.D. "The Genetical Theory of Social Behaviour." Journal of Theoretical Biology 7, 1 (1964): 1-52.

Ohnuki-Tierney, Emiko. "An Octopus Headache? A Lamprey Boil? Multi-sensory Perception of 'Habitual Illness' and World View of Ainu." Journal of Anthropological Research 33, 3 (1977): 245-257.

Polgar, Steven. "Health and Human Behavior: Areas of Interest Common to the Social and Medical Sciences." Current Anthropology 3, 2 (1962): 159.

McCullough, John M. "Human Ecology, Heat Adaptation, and Belief Systems: The Hot-Cold Syndrome of Yucatan." Journal of Anthropological Research 29 (1973): 32-36.

van den Bergh, Pierre L. and David P. Barash. "Inclusive Fitness and Human Family Structure." The American Anthropologist 79, 4 (December, 1977): 809-823.

Wynne-Edwards, V.C. Animal Dispersion in Relation to Social Behaviour. Edinburgh: Oliver and Boyd, 1962.

5. The Influence of Psychosocial Factors on Susceptibility to Physical Illness

The primary assumption in assigning a role to psychosocial factors in disease susceptibility is that, given a reasonably large sample of persons all of whom are equally exposed to a particular pathogen or disease-causing vector, some will become sick sooner, some will become sick later, some will experience the illness in severe form, others will become only mildly sick, and still others will not develop the illness at all. This is more than an assumption; it is an observation, and it expresses the concept of individual differences in disease susceptibility: differences in susceptibility to illness generally, and differences in susceptibility to specific ailments. As efforts have been made to analyze the origins and nature of these variations in individual susceptibility, three classes of factors have been differentiated: (1) constitutional; (2) situational; and (3) psychological. Constitutional factors are those of heredity and early perinatal conditions which provide a friendly or antagonistic biological substrate for support of the disease process. Situational factors are conditions of the environment which alter the level of the individual's natural resistance; these may be physical or psychological in nature. My focus is on the latter, and specifically on those aspects of the individual's life situation which are perceived by him or her in such a fashion that they create internal tension. To the outside observer, the individual's situation may be seen as one which is stressful, but what is critical is whether or not an individual experiences the situation as one of demands or threats which exceed his or her usual coping capacities. When this is true, the result is internalized tension which reduces the adaptive flexibility of physiological responses, and hence lowers the threshold of resistance, or increases the susceptibility to disease. The constitutional factors are essentially fixed or stable for the individual, as is his or her status with respect to proper immunization against common diseases. The situational

factors are obviously variable, and the psychological factors
even more so. Psychosocial factors may be defined as those
aspects of the individual's life situation which have a high
content of intrapersonal and interpersonal significance, are
closely entailed in meeting basic roles in family and community, and carry broad markers of "success" or "failure,"
thus being tied to morale or self-esteem. The individual's
disease susceptibility is a fluctuating index which varies
over time as a complex function of the interaction of the
constitutional, situational, and psychological dimensions.
If we conceive of disease susceptibility as a fluctuating index of this nature, we can readily understand two aspects of
the current state of knowledge about the role of psychosocial
factors in susceptibility to disease: (1) Looked at as a
single variable, indices of situational stress show only a
low, albeit statistically reliable, degree of association
with the incidence of physical disease, rarely accounting for
more than 10% of the variance (Rabkin and Streuning, 1976).
(2) When groups of individuals are identified by a personality typology as being at "high risk" for coronary disease
and followed to discover the subsequent incidence of actual
illness, the false positive rate approaches 25% (Rosenman,
Brand, Jenkins, et al., 1975). These two findings point the
direction for needed research: Ceteris is never paribus,
and we must look at multiple variables in designs that take
interrelationships into account.

In the last three to four decades, there has been an up-
surge in research directed to the thesis, in broadest terms,
that how people live determines how they die. More precisely, the general hypothesis under investigation is: Given
exposure to a pathogenic agent, individuals are more or less
predisposed to become ill as a function of their psychological histories. With presence of pathogenic vectors a given
or constant, certain aspects of daily life constitute "risk
factors" which may increase the likelihood of illness.
Broadly conceived, so-called psychological "risk factors"
are conceptualized under two major rubrics: (1) stress, or
stressors; and (2) life styles or personality.

From a public health point of view, there is a paradox:
medical science and technology, through eradication of
plague, discovery of antibiotics, and other breakthroughs,
has increased longevity, but men and women are dying or being
incapacitated prematurely as a result of behaviors which may
be viewed as subtly (or not so subtly) self-destructive, or
as a function of life circumstances which impair their natural resistance to disease. It can be said, ironically, of
many cardiac patients, "They haven't the heart to go on living!"

The hard research to discover psychosocial precursors as necessary, if not sufficient, causal factors in physical illness is new. The general concepts on which these studies rest are almost as old as the history of medicine itself. The ancients spoke of "Mens sana in corpore sano," a healthy mind in a healthy body. But the equation is reversible. Modern medicine has come to an appreciation that a healthy body requires a healthy mind. Mind and body are very useful abstractions, but the inescapable fact is that the human being is one: an organismic, holistic, integrated, unified field of continuous energy exchange between the "poles" of the "psyche" and the "soma."

We are moving toward an increasingly refined understanding of the continuity of the person-environment interaction and of the feedback loops of the neuro-endocrine system whereby, for example, the perception of stress may be adapted to by an increase in blood pressure, and the formal diagnosis of hypertension may be perceived as further stress, and so on. We are a far step from the priest-physicians of old when we can assign a numerical index to the amount of adaptation-demanding change in life situation experienced by an individual in the previous six months or year; and when we can, with substantial reliability, assign a person to a type B personality classification. Certainly these are more operationally satisfying maneuvers than to speak of the unkindness of the gods or an excess of bile. But how far we still are from where we wish to be!

It has long been obvious that serious physical illness can give rise to emotional disturbance, to personality disruption, to impaired psychological functions, especially to anxiety and depression. Increasingly, we are coming to see that the way individuals perceive and interpret their environment, and the decisions they make as to how to cope with that perceived environment, leads to behaviors which may have profound implications for their physical health. Consider a generally accepted causal chain: stress leads to tension; tension leads to learned tension-relieving behaviors, e.g., smoking and drinking; and these behaviors may lead to cancer and general physical debilitation.

For many individuals in our fast-paced, impersonal, technological, production and achievement oriented culture, it may be said that the physical-social environment is stressful. But not all individuals experience such an environment as stressful, at least to a degree that generates chronic and high levels of tension. A necessary intervening variable is the perception (the interpretation, the construction, the introjection) of that environment as stressful.

It is the manner of perception, the work of the mind, that provides the psychosocial matrix for stress-induced upheavals in the individual's total functioning : "One man's meat is another man's poison." Some persons thrive on pressure and cannot (or will not?) function without it. Others, in the same situation, facing the same demands, develop ulcers.

Extensive physiological research (Selye, 1956, and others) has demonstrated the health damaging consequences of chronically high demand for adaptive responses at the level of organ systems. Psychological and sociological research have demonstrated that chains of situational experiences and characterological variables are reliably associated with susceptibility to physical illnesses.

Beginning in the late 1960's with the innovative studies of Holmes and Rahe, there has been a progression of studies which demonstrate that both the occurrence of illness and the severity of illness are reliably associated with significant changes in the general life situation of patients in the immediate pre-morbid period. The generality of their findings has been given significant support through cross-cultural validation (Holmes and Rahe, 1969; Wyler, Masuda, and Holmes, 1971; Theorell and Rahe, 1971).

Hinkle (1974) and his colleagues, in a series of studies which nicely combine clinical and epidemiological methods, have demonstrated the manner in which the interaction of personality and psychosocial history variables serves as potentiators or inhibitors in determining whether environmental/situational factors will give rise to physical illness.

The Western Collaborative Group Study, under the leadership of Rosenman and Friedman, has produced striking evidence that certain personality variables play a contributory role not only in the occurrence of coronary disease, but in severity and susceptibility to recurrence (Rosenman and Friedman, 1960; Rosenman, Brand, Jenkins, et al., 1975).

These two broad lines of research on situational stress and personality typology in relation to physical illness represent persistent, programmatic endeavors with extensive cross-validation. Investigation of psychosocial variables in other illnesses, notably cancer, is also being pursued, but with less standardization of methodology and instrumentation (Bahnson, 1969).

The accumulated research to date on psychosocial factors in disease susceptibility has served to validate the crude

formulations of the past. The generation of our forebears
would say, "He became ill as a result of overwork," or "She
has a nervous stomach." The studies of physiologists, epidemiologists, psychologists, sociologists, anthropologists,
and physicians have established that there <u>is</u> an association
between life experiences or situational stress and susceptibility to physical illness. And they have established that
there is an association between certain personality types or
temperaments and susceptibility to illness. But the level of
association is one of probability, and low probability at
that. Our goal is to be able to identify the <u>individual</u> at
high risk so that, hopefully, we can take steps that will reduce that risk.

Those researchers who have established that illness susceptibility is increased with increased frequency or severity
of change in the life situation have moved us along. They
have provided a basis for identifying samples of high risk
persons for prospective studies so that we can look more
closely for those variables which seem to differentiate those
who succumb from those who do not, since membership in a high
risk group per se does not yield practical prediction.

Those researchers who have delineated the personality
type with a high susceptibility to coronary heart disease
have likewise made possible the identification of false posi-
tives. And, again, by careful comparative, prospective scru-
tiny of those who succumb and those who do not, we can move
gradually to an increasing understanding of the interaction
between environment, perception, temperament, and physical
breakdown.

We have a fairly good grasp of the sort of changes in
individuals' life situations which are likely to prove
stressful and increase disease susceptibility. Also, we can
fairly reliably identify individuals whose life style can be
characterized by a relatively high level of chronic and
largely self-induced tension. We need to study in depth the
interaction between situational crisis and life style as they
relate to disease history. The situational stress lines of
research and the personality typing researches need to be
brought together. This will be done most effectively when
we recognize that it is the way in which individuals inte-
grate their <u>perception of their situation</u> and <u>their perceptions of themselves</u> which determines greater or lesser resistance to physical illness. Psychosocial stressors are
not inherently causal, but onlly potentially so, as are variables of temperament and emotionality. It is the way in which
the interplay of these two dimensions affects the behavior of
individuals that influences their susceptibility. Their

health-neglecting or health-sustaining behaviors are crucial. For example, the Type A personality (the hard-driving, compulsive, time sensitive, restless, aggressive individual), confronted by the situational change of a significant promotion or occupational advancement, may celebrate by joining an exclusive athletic club and put into his weekly schedule two or three hours of vigorous physical exercise, previously absent, and thus enhance his overall health. Or he may join the same club and substitute a two or three martini, high calorie lunch for his previous soup or sandwich diet, increasing his weight and impairing his health. There are psychological determinants of which pattern he adopts. The same "high risk" individual in personality terms becomes, with one adjustment to change, less susceptible, and, with another, more susceptible. Faced with an increase in situational demand or environmental stress, the Type A person, if he or she is a smoker, may increase the use of cigarettes, with implications for subsequent health. But if he or she is a non-smoker, this will not happen. Consider a woman who experiences a sudden significant emotional loss, e.g., death of a spouse. A period of grief, mourning, and depression is likely; and a common symptom of depression is loss of appetite and reduced food intake. If it happens that this individual was significantly overweight, it may be that the period of emotional dysphoria, when over, will find her with a better state of physical health! A paradox! All this is by way of saying that the promising lines of research into the relationships of life experience and personality to disease susceptibility must be pursued in the direction of increasing specificity of variables. Accuracy of prediction will be increased as we increase the number of cells in our actuarial tables, with each cell representing accumulated experience as to the disease history of a sufficiently large sample of persons who are homogeneous for a large number of relevant variables. Still other personality constellations may become reliably associated with gastrointestinal susceptibility, with neuromuscular disorders, with illnesses of the respiratory system, etc.

The current methods of deriving an index of an individual's stress level have been criticized on a number of grounds, e.g., that they lack homogeneous content and include both "desirable" and "undesirable" life situation changes, such as death of a close relative and achievement of a special award or recognition. If stress is a unitary factor, and if there are no significant differences in the adaptive response to "good" stress versus "bad" stress, then such lumping of qualitatively different changes in life situation will be justified. But this is a significant empiri-

cal question which deserves careful study (Rabkin and
Struening, 1976).

With the translation of the indicators originally based
on clinical examination and interview into structured perfor-
mance tests and questionnaires suitable for self-report,
there is now available a method for objective and reliable
screening of large numbers of persons and their assignment to
a personality classification, such as a Type A or Type B
(Bortner and Rosenman, 1967; Jenkins, Rosenman, and Friedman, 1967). Validation of such classifications against external criteria, particularly to provide concurrent validation, cannot be foregone. It must be recognized that the
personality picture of a coronary patient may be only a partially accurate picture of pre-morbid character, and that the
fact of serious illness is likely to create distortions in
self-report. The methods for achieving increased reliability
and validity with these basically diagnostic problems are
well known and can yield improved measures. Significant
progress is less dependent upon refinements in these methodologies than it is upon research designs which permit analyses
of the complex interrelationships between life experiences,
immediate situational stress, established behavior patterns
(or personality), and the threshold susceptibility to particular illness which is established by constitutional predisposition, or "somatic compliance." In studying the role of
psychosocial factors in illness, we can probably learn as
much through careful study of "resistant" individuals as in
investigation of the "susceptibles." Many of the crucial
questions as to the relationship between psychosocial factors
and susceptibility will only be answered with the application
of these measures in prospective studies of large samples of
persons who are initially free of disease.

If the yield to date in terms of formulations and pre-
dictions from psychosocial factors is at best heuristic and
propadeutic, we are none the less indebted to those pioneer
researchers, Cannon, Meyer, Selye, Dunbar, Hinkle, Holmes
and Rahe, Friedman and Rosenman, Jenkins, who have moved
medicine significantly toward a conception that all illness
is somatopsychic.

References

Bahnson, C.B., ed. "Second Conference on Psychophysiological Aspects of Cancer." Annals of the New York Academy of Sciences, 164 (1969), 307-364.

Bortner, R.W. and R.H. Rosenman. "The Measurement of Pattern A Behavior." J. Chronic. Dis., 20 (1967), 525-533.

Dohrenwend, B.S. and B.P. Dohrenwend, eds. Stressful Life Events: Their Nature and Effects. New York: John Wiley & Sons, 1974.

Dunbar, Flanders. Emotions and Bodily Changes (4th edition). New York: Columbia University Press, 1954.

Engel, George L. "The Need for a New Medical Model: A Challenge for Biomedicine." Science, 196 (1977), 129-136.

Epstein, Frederick H. "The Epidemiology of Coronary Heart Disease." J. Chron. Dis., 18 (1965), 735-774.

Friedman, Meyer. Pathogenesis of Coronary Heart Disease. New York: McGraw-Hill, 1969.

Hinkle, Lawrence E. "The Effect of Exposure to Culture Change, Social Change, and Changes in Interpersonal Relationships on Health." Chapter 2, pp. 9-44, in Dohrenwend and Dohrenwend, op. cit.

Holmes, T.H. and R.H. Rahe. "The Social Readjustment Rating Scale." J. Psychosom. Res., 11 (1969), 213-218.

Jenkins, C.D., R.H. Rosenman, and M. Friedman. "Development of an Objective Psychological Test for the Determination of the Coronary-Prone Behavior Pattern in Employed Men." J. Chronic Dis., 20 (1967), 371-379.

Jenkins, C.D., R.H. Rosenman, and M. Friedman. "Replicability of Rating of the Coronary Prone Behavior Pattern." Br. J. Prev. Soc. Med., 225 (1969), 237-244.

Jenkins, C. David. "Psychological and Social Precursors of Coronary Disease." New England J. Med., 284 (1971), 244-255, 307-317.

Rabkin, J.G. and E.L. Streuning. "Life Events, Stress, and Illness." Science, 194 (1976), 1013-1020.

Rosenman, R.H. and M. Friedman. "Overt Behavior Pattern in Coronary Heart Disease." J. Amer. Med. Assoc., 173 (1960), 1320.

Rosenman, R.H., M. Friedman, R. Strauss, et al. "Coronary Heart Disease in the Western Collaborative Group Study: A Follow-up Experience of Two Years." J. Amer. Med. Assoc., 195 (1966), 130-136.

Rosenman, R.H., R.J. Brand, C.D. Jenkins, et al. "Coronary Heart Disease in the Western Collaborative Group Study: Final Follow-up Experience of 8½ Years." J. Amer. Med. Assoc., 233 (1975), 872-877.

Schwartz, G.E. and S.M. Weiss, eds. Yale Conference on Behavioral Medicine. February, 1977. Proceedings. National Heart, Lung and Blood Institute.

Selye, Hans. The Stress of Life. New York: McGraw-Hill, 1956.

Theorell, T. and R.H. Rahe. "Psychosocial Factors and Myocardial Infarction: I. An Inpatient Study in Sweden." J. Psychosom. Res., 15 (1971), 25-31.

Weiss, Stephen M., ed. Proceedings of the National Heart and Lung Institute Working Conference on Health Behavior. May 12-15, 1975 DHEW Publication No. (NIH) 76-868.

Wyler, A.R., M. Masuda, and T.H. Holmes. "Magnitude of Life Events and Seriousness of Illness." Psychosom. Med., 33 (1971), 115-122.

6. Sociocultural and Psychological Aspects of the Utilization of Health Services

This paper seeks to assess contributions of behavioral scientists to our understanding of sociocultural and psychological factors as these relate to health care utilization. Relevant research and theory will be critically reviewed with a focus on areas of current research interest. The discussion will center on acute medical services provided by physicians on an ambulatory basis, but most issues raised and conclusions drawn are applicable to other areas of health care utilization. Particular note will be made of areas and issues, both substantive and methodological, which appear particularly promising for future investigation.

Most of the research in this area grows out of two concerns. First, beginning in the early 1930's with the first survey research work in health care utilization, there developed an awareness of the unequal distribution of the use of health services by persons in various social and economic groups (Falk et al., 1933; Zborowski, 1952; Saunders, 1954, Clark, 1959). There was considerable concern that certain groups, including the poor, culturally and ethnically segregated (Mexican-Americans, recent European immigrants, etc.), and Blacks, were not receiving their "fair" share of the benefits made available through the rapid growth and increasing sophistication of modern scientific medicine. Second, with the introduction of Medicaid and Medicare programs and other public financing of health care, the percent of total expenditures on health care contributed from public sources rose precipitously during the late 1960's (Cooper, 1969). In the face of what was seen by many as a financial crisis, research attention became heavily focused on issues related to "overutilization" and "improper" care.

Thus, research in health care utilization focused on social and cultural variables as sources of inequitable and insufficient care in early years, while attention in more recent years has focused more heavily on financial issues and concerns with inappropriate and unnecessary health care utilization. Currently, I feel there is an increased interest again in psychological and sociocultural issues.

Proper Health Care Utilization

Research has shown large differences in the patterns of health care utilization across countries and within regions. Rates of hospitalization in some countries are over twice as high as what they are in others (Anderson and Sheatsley, 1967) and rates of physician visits are several times higher in certain countries or regions of countries than in others (Shuval, 1970). These differences cannot be explained by differences in known morbidity rates or demographic characteristics of populations being served (Anderson and Andersen, 1972: 390). As Anderson and Sheatsley (1967: 4) observed with regard to hospital utilization, "the obvious conclusion is that the volume of 'proper' hospital care is highly elastic, so elastic that the generalization can be made that there is no 'proper' level of use of hospital care; there is no generally accepted standard." "Standards of medical care can be as subjective as proper standards for food, clothing, and shelter" (Anderson and Sheatsley, 1967: 5).

There are no "medical-scientific" standards by which a proper level of care can be clearly ascertained. Practitioners themselves differ on the proper utilization patterns appropriate to various medical conditions and often disagree on whether certain complaints, such as psychological or personal problems, are appropriate subjects for our medical care system.

Certain researchers, nevertheless, still proceed as if social and cultural factors are confounding issues that lead to inappropriate utilization of health facilities (cf. Restuccia and Holloway, 1976), rather than factors that shape perceptions of what is proper care. Specifically, what is "proper" care differs from one person to the next due to social and psychological factors, and patients' views may differ from physicians'. If social and psychological variations are acknowledged by the practitioner or administrator, then a key question becomes how the practitioner or administrator can be responsive to a particular patient's perceived needs as well as to the practitioner's professional judgment of what the patient should receive.

Complexities in the Concept of Utilization

The variety of types of care must be recognized in
health care utilization research. Physician care may be by
a general practitioner or specialist. Physicians may be consulted in their offices, over the telephone, in hospital
wards, or in emergency rooms. Hospital utilization varies by
number of admissions, length of stay, and type of admission
(elective or nonelective).

Both within and outside of physicians' offices and hospitals, a variety of health care related professionals practice. Psychologists, social workers, physician assistants,
and nurses all serve as primary care providers within our
health care system (Guillozet, 1975; Fink, 1969). In addition, dental care is often highly differentiated from general
medical care. Comparison across medical care systems can be
difficult because providers of services are often not easily
equated, as in the case of physicians in the United States as
compared to physicians in Poland (Bice and White, 1971).

Within each of these types of providers and settings, a
variety of types of services may be rendered, and each of
these services may be influenced by various factors. While
the largest type of service is care of somatic complaints,
such complaints may be variously used: for instance, as a
means of establishing a relationship with the physician for
the underlying purpose of dealing with social or personal
problems (Balint, 1957). Understanding treatment of somatic
complaints may be further complicated because patterns of use
may vary by whether the complaint is presented during an initial visit by a patient, a followup visit to receive continued care, or a referral from one part of the health care system to another (Bice and White, 1971). Preventive health behavior may itself be variously motivated, as when prenatal
care is engaged in as a condition of receipt of maternity
benefits (McKinlay, 1972) or when physical checkups are used
as a means of bringing acute somatic complaints to a physician (Kasl, 1974). In addition, preventive health behavior
such as physical checkups may be disguised as symptomatic
problems for purposes of insurance reimbursement or obtaining early access to physician care. Thus, a type of health
care utilization, such as a visit to a physician's office,
may consist of any of several rather distinct utilization
phenomena.

Too narrow a perspective on health care utilization may
also lead to overlooking related health care services such as
nursing home care, podiatrist services, opthalmologists' visits, and chiropractic adjustments. Also, a variety of health

related or alternative services may be chosen by a particular individual in lieu of physician care. These may include generally accepted sources such as school nurses and public health nurses, but they may also include sources of advice such as faith healers or Scientologists.

Health care utilization need not be measured with regard to specific individuals, but can be considered on a family basis (Fink, 1969; Andersen, 1968). Also, the fact that parents structure the health care utilization of children indicates that child health care utilization is a distinct category and needs to be studied as such. A major limitation of health care utilization research to this point is the failure to sufficiently focus on these unique types of utilization, and a major potential and possibility for the future concerns these various distinctions, especially the types of services and providers beyond those normally considered as the core of our health care system.

Dangers of Aggregating Heterogeneous Utilization Measures

Kalimo et al. (1972) report data from a cross-national study which indicates that various types of health care utilization are correlated at only a low level (measures of types of utilization shared only between one and two percent of their variance). The patterns of correlation between types of health care utilization were similar from one area to another in countries, but there was little pattern found between countries. Andersen (1968: 29-30) reports somewhat moderate although higher levels of association between several types of utilization (hospitalization, physician visits, drug use, dental visits) by families, and concludes "Families who are large consumers of one service are not necessarily large consumers of another" (the average Pearsonian correlation among these utilization measures was .20). It is not surprising, then, that efforts to predict health care utilization measures that are aggregates of these largely independent phenomena have not been promising. Andersen (1968: 21-30) has made one of the most extensive and well known attempts to aggregate health care utilization data into a single index. His attempt has been criticized as being insufficiently attentive to differences between these types of care and the real possibility that types of care may have substantially different predictors (Kirscht, 1974: 396; Hershey et al., 1975: 838; Welch et al., 1973). An increasingly frequent observation and critique is that progress in understanding health care utilization has been hindered by research focusing on types of utilization which were comprised of heterogeneous categories of utilization (Kasl, 1974: 437;

Bice and White, 1971: 257;   Kalimo et al., 1972). Research focusing on certain more specific types of utilization, such as preventive dental care, suggest that ability to understand and predict types of health care utilization may be aided by a focus on more specific types of behavior, defined both in terms of type of service, motivation, and the point in a series of contacts, e.g., initial contact, followup, or referral (Bice and White, 1971: 257).

Review of this complex medical care system and the multiple ways in which it is used makes it clear that this paper cannot reasonably hope to even touch on each of these various possibilities. We will focus our discussion largely on ambulatory use of physician services for acute care because this is an area in which there is considerable research interest, increasing utilization and costs (Anderson and Andersen, 1972), and a substantial degree of discretion exercised on the part of patients.

Theories of Health Care Utilization

No overall theory of health care utilization, or even a limited theory of utilization of physician services, exists (Greenlick et al., 1968; Anderson and Andersen, 1972: 386-387). A number of reviews and discussions of various models are available (McKinlay, 1972; Anderson and Bartkus, 1973; McKinlay and Dutton, 1974; Kirscht, 1974; Becker et al., 1977).

Decision Points or Stage Models

A number of available "models" of utilization of physician services are built on the notion of stages or decision points (see Suchman, 1965a; Fabrega, 1973). For example, Zola (1964) notes five types of "cues" in a patient's decision to seek medical care: (1) an "interpersonal crisis" that calls attention to the patient's symptoms, (2) social interference in social activities by symptoms, (3) sanctioning of the symptom by significant others who tell the person to seek care, (4) a threat to vocational activities, and (5) a comparison of symptoms with those experienced earlier by self or friends. Five stages or decision points are outlined by Kadushin (1958-1959) in his model of decision making with regard to undertaking psychotherapy. These are recognition of the emotional problem, exposure to the existence of a problem with a circle of friends and relatives, a decision to seek professional help, a selection of a professional area of help, and a selection of a specific practitioner.

"Sets of Variables" Models

Several other "models" provide what are essentially variables or sets of variables which may be useful predictors of utilization. Andersen (1968) suggests a health care utilization model with three segments: (1) a predisposition to use service; (2) enabling factors or means to secure services; and (3) a perceived need for service. Mechanic (1968) lists a series of ten different factors which may affect utilization of physician services (see also Mechanic, 1962).

The Health Belief Model described variables useful in explaining preventive health behaviors (Rosenstock, 1966), and has since been applied to illness behavior (Kirscht, 1974). The model focuses on the readiness of an individual to use medical services, e.g., perceived vulnerability from illness, the perceived consequences of certain illnesses, the perceived benefits of health care, the perceived barriers to taking action, and the notion that utilization may require a cue or trigger for action. The utility of this model as applied to acute care rather than preventive situations has been questioned (Becker et al., 1977: 29-30).

There has been little "causal" modeling of data. This lack of causal modeling, including a search for intervening variables to explain more antecedent ones, may in part be due to a lack of sufficiently well developed theory, but it is also due to a lack of strong predictors of utilization behaviors which could be the basis of useful modeling (see Roghmann, 1975a: 122).

Limitations, Possibilities and Alternatives

Both the stage model presented by Fabrega (1973) and the Health Belief Model (Kirscht, 1974) assume a "rational" calculating man who weighs the costs and benefits of care. Roghmann and Haggerty (1975: 152-153) argue that a different emphasis may be useful.

First, we think of illness behavior as impulsive rather than planned. The recognition that an individual's coping abilities have been exceeded triggers his behavior if care is available. Second, illness behavior is perceived of as a short-term process, where timing is of greater importance than the decision itself. This combination of impulsive behavior occurring in a short-term process gives, over the long run, the impression of randomness.

They see the Health Belief Model as too "rational, goal directed, and imbedded in long-term planning" (Roghmann and Haggerty, 1975: 153). Some of the frustration and lack of success in finding substantial predictors of utilization of physician services through survey interviews may be because survey interviews are power instruments to capture the more immediate aspects of a person's situation and a specific timing and context of it. This "situational" perspective has not been developed even into a nascent model; and, despite the apparent difficulties, it may be possible to specify some of the situational contexts and personal characteristics associated even with "impulsive" behavior.

Different types of models would need to be developed for different types, not only of dependent variables, but of independent variables as well. Greenlick et al. (1968) suggest that different factors may affect different types of health care utilization, depending on the type of disease. They suggest that theoretical and empirical models be built separately for different disease categories. The utility of this approach is unknown, but several studies have found that, for different groups, e.g., income or racial groups, different variables predict utilization.

While the existing models are numerous and often extensive, there are several areas in which theoretical work has not progressed far and in which there is likely to be considerable potential. First, none of the models deals adequately with the possible choice of alternative services. The theories are generally built on the assumption that a person will choose to use typical medical services or none at all, with the possible exception of self care or self medication. However, it is increasingly clear that persons use a variety of types of care when faced with a potential medical problem (Greenley and Mechanic, 1976a). Second, these models are substantially deficient in their incorporation of variables related to the services provided. In particular, they fail to develop the place or importance of past experiences with physicians in general or with particular physicians in the decision to use care (cf. McKinlay, 1972). Third, models are needed which take into account issues related to chronic illness as distinguished from acute care issues (Kasl, 1974: 447-448). Fourth, an important area which has received only minor attention concerns the socialization of health beliefs and behaviors during childhood (cf. Mechanic, 1964). It may be very difficult to develop an adequate understanding of health care utilization without further knowledge in this area of childhood socialization and health. Fifth, these models are inadequately developed with regard to what Freidson (1961) has called the lay referral system. This is the

notion that persons consult with family and friends before
seeking professional help; more theoretical and empirical
work is certainly needed in this area (Kasl, 1974: 447;
Robinson, 1971).

Sociodemographic Correlates of Physician Visits

Early behavioral science research into health care utilization revealed differential utilization of health care in
various social and demographic groups. Most of the subsequent research by behavioral scientists in health care utilization can be conceptualized as a search for variables which
would help to explain the differential rates of health care
utilization across these various social groups (McKinlay,
1972: 121-122). It is not our purpose here to review this
literature regarding sociodemographic correlates of health
care utilization; reviews of this literature are available
(Aday and Eichhorn, 1972; Anderson and Andersen, 1972). In
general, use of physicians' services is greater by females
than males, and utilization rates are higher among the very
young and the elderly segments of the population. Persons
of Jewish religiocultural backgrounds have been found to
have consistently higher rates of health care utilization,
including use of physician services. Persons with more formal education are usually found to have higher rates of physician visits. Most studies have shown that persons with
higher incomes have greater levels of utilization, but more
recent studies suggest this gap is narrowing or may have, in
some instances, disappeared (Galvin and Fan, 1975; Salber et
al., 1976).

Behavioral science researchers are increasingly aware
that these relationships may be changing over time. For instance, Roghmann (1975b: 199) finds that utilization of physicians by children has been dropping in recent years, while
others, using a similar measure, have reported an increase
in use of physician services by the adult population (Anderson and Andersen, 1972). As these changes are observed, the
task of the behavioral science researcher becomes increasingly difficult. Theories must take into account dynamic as
well as static situations, and monitoring of relationships
must be continued.

It must be noted that the data on which these generali-
zations are based concern the United States. Bice et al.
(1972), in their multinational study of health care utilization, found that relationships between utilization rates and
sociodemographic variables are different in various national
health care systems. For example, they found that income was
directly related to use of physician services in only

one-half of the countries they studied. Thus, these relationships between sociodemographic factors and utilization rates may be due to variations in health care systems as much as in the types of people using them.

In almost no case do these sociodemographic variables explain a substantial amount of the variance in use of physician services. An adequate understanding of health care utilization must go well beyond being able to account empirically or theoretically for these relationships.

Morbidity and Utilization

Differences in morbidity may account for some or all of the differences in use of physician services by persons in these various sociodemographic groups. Perceived morbidity is strongly related to, and is probably the strongest predictor of, use of physician services (Hulka et al., 1972; Gaspard and Hopkins, 1967; Galvin and Fan, 1975; Bice and White, 1969; Hershey et al., 1975; Andersen, 1968). It may seem only common sense that persons reporting more symptoms, diseases, and conditions would make greater use of physician services. Yet symptoms are very pervasive in populations (Hammond, 1964; Andersen et al., 1968). Many more people report symptomatic conditions than seek physician aid for them, and people clearly report symptoms for which they do not seek treatment (Hyman, 1970).

Because reported symptoms are powerful predictors of health care utilization and are important concerns in their own right, considerable empirical and theoretical effort has been made to understand the social and psychological factors affecting their recognition and expression. It is useful to distinguish three types of effort in this regard. First is the effort to examine the awareness or realization by an individual of the presence of an abnormal bodily state. Second is the investigation of how an individual comes to attribute meaning to a bodily state such that it comes to be seen as an indication of illness. Third are efforts to assess the quality or nature of abnormal bodily states already defined as symptoms of illness as these relate to utilization decisions. Each of these requires separate discussion, for each poses separate problems and possibilities for research.

Awareness of Abnormal Bodily States

The first and possibly the most difficult and problematic area concerns how individuals come to realize they have abnormal bodily states. Laboratory studies on pain and drugs designed to alleviate pain clearly suggest that the social

context and psychological orientations of persons are critical to their perception and recognition of physical trauma
as painful (Mechanic, 1972a, 1972b). Pain medications, for
instance, that have been shown effective in relieving pain in
clinical settings have been much less effective in changing
perceptions of pain in laboratory situations. In these laboratory situations, persons may not experience similar pain
from similar trauma because the trauma is expected and interpreted as part of an experimental situation. Persons at
lower socioeconomic levels have been reported to be less
likely to think of themselves as tired than are persons be-
longing to upper social classes because tiredness may be less
often an unusual bodily state for individuals of low social
class (Robinson, 1971). Chronic conditions are often not reported by individuals when interviewed about their symptoms
about "sickness" or "illness", possibly because they are not
seen as "unusual" bodily states but rather as "typical"
(Robinson, 1971). Clark (1959) reports that Mexican-Americans often did not take their children to physicians for care
of diarrhea because diarrhea was such a prevalent condition
among children in that subcultural group that it was not considered abnormal.

Signs and conditions may come to be seen as abnormal
bodily states at times of heightened sensitivity to bodily
conditions. Stress has been noted as a possible cause for
heightened sensitivity and the production of an awareness of
conditions already present (Kasl and Cobb, 1966). Zola
(1964) suggests that an "interpersonal crisis" may trigger
recognition of an abnormal bodily state or symptom. Psychological distress may be related to greater sensitivity to
symptoms or greater reporting of them (Tessler and Mechanic,
1978). The process of recognition is difficult to study with
current prevalent survey research methodologies which rely on
the reports of symptoms by individuals who are already aware
of their conditions as abnormal bodily states. Thus, I feel
that this area is substantially under-researched and of potentially great promise in our understanding of health care
utilization.

Illness Attributions

Factors affecting the likelihood of interpreting an abnormal bodily state as a symptomatic condition connoting illness include a variety of possibly overlapping factors.
First, a person is assumed to be more likely to assess his
"phenomenological experience" as an indication of an illness
condition if he evaluates it negatively (Fabrega, 1973).
Certain abnormal bodily states may be sought and valued positively, such as experiences with marijuana (Becker, 1963).

Second, it may be likely that a bodily state is seen as an illness indication if a high value is placed on being well (McKinlay and Dutton, 1974). Third, persons are sometimes seen as having a variety of available nonillness attributions which they can use to make sense out of a particular bodily experience (Scheff, 1966). For instance, Suchman (1965a: 118) found that 13% of persons experiencing symptoms initially attributed them to tension or the weather, even though the symptoms subsequently led to their hospitalization or bed-disability. Research in this area has been limited by the tendency for health care researchers to focus on symptom experiences of individuals rather than on bodily states which may or may not be seen as symptomatic of illness conditions. Given the high prevalence of symptomatic conditions and experiences of various bodily states, it may be critical to our understanding of the use of physician services to further explore this area.

Assessments of Symptoms

Most commonly, researchers have queried people concerning their symptoms and then proceeded to link various evaluations of these symptomatic conditions to use of physician services. Assessment of seriousness of symptoms has been most commonly researched. Hulka et al. (1972) interviewed people about their symptoms during the four weeks prior to the interview and then had them assess the seriousness of these symptoms. Symptom seriousness measured in this way was strongly related to physician visits (see also Suchman, 1965a: 121). Anderson and Sheatsley (1967) found 79% of symptomatic people to have delayed seeking care because they assessed these symptoms as not serious or as likely to go away by themselves.

Other factors that have been suggested or researched in connection with symptom assessment include duration of the symptom (Hulka et al., 1972; Mechanic, 1968), impingement of the symptom on vocational or social role functioning (Zola, 1964; Fabrega, 1973; Suchman, 1965a), the familiarity of the symptom to the person (Mechanic, 1968, 1972a; Zola, 1964), feelings of risk or vulnerability caused by the symptom (Mechanic, 1972a), and whether the symptom causes "worry" or emotional distress (Hulka et al., 1972). These factors are not necessarily conceptually distinct nor are they exhaustive of all possibilities which have been suggested or researched. The category of seriousness of symptoms, which has been most clearly shown to be related to use of physician services, possibly incorporates assessments by individuals of the impingement upon their role functioning, the duration of the symptoms, the risk posed by the symptoms as they assess it, and so forth.

These aspects of symptom assessment have been most commonly measured in retrospective interview studies. As such, the assessment of the symptom may be highly colored by the experience that the person had when taking the symptom to a physician. Symptoms taken to a physician may come to be seen as more consequential and symptoms not taken may be minimized or even forgotten for various psychological reasons. There is, therefore, serious question that symptom assessments cause utilization and not <u>vice versa</u>.

Symptom experience and reporting of symptoms have been shown to be related to sociodemographic factors, and this may help explain the relationship between sociodemographic variables and physician visits. Suchman (1965a: 119) argues that women and older people take symptoms more seriously. Various studies have linked ethnic and religiocultural groups to differential assessment of symptom experiences (Zborowski, 1952; Zola, 1966, 1964; Mechanic, 1963; Guttmacher and Elinson, 1971). While it is not clear how socioeconomic status relates to the perception and experience of symptoms (Mechanic, 1969), various studies have reported relationships between aspects of symptom assessment and socioeconomic status. Lower socioeconomic status groups may be less likely to deem their symptoms serious (Koos, 1954); may have an equal likelihood of interpreting bodily symptoms as illness, while at the same time having more incapacitation (Suchman, 1965a: 119); and may under-report morbidity in surveys (Mechanic, 1968). Thus issues of symptom recognition, attribution, and assessment are related to several sociodemographic factors and may help to explain the relationships of certain sociodemographic factors and utilization.

Income and Utilization

As noted above, income differences in rates of physician utilization and other types of medical care are narrowing and may have largely disappeared. Health care utilization researchers need to fully recognize that income related inequities still exist for certain populations and that those inequities may persist due to other non-financial social and psychological reasons.

For low income persons paying for their care, cost is still a major determinant in use of services (Hershey et al., 1975: 845; Bice et al., 1973) and copayments on insurance coverage may have a substantial inhibiting effect on use of services (Roemer et al., 1975: 457-458; Newhouse et al., 1974). In a study by Anderson and Sheatsley (1967), 3% of persons reporting symptoms delayed seeking care due to cost; Suchman (1965a: 120) found that, of people reporting symptoms serious enough to require hospitalization or bed-disability days, 8% waited before seeking care due to financial reasons. These differences in utilization by cost of care and income are in increasing danger of being ignored in light of the gross statistics on equalization of utilization by income groups. Physician utilization among low income people may not now differ substantially across income groups. Yet, within low income groups, recipients of, for instance, Medicaid have relatively high levels of physician utilization, and those not insured or covered under a public program have relatively low rates (NCHS, 1972; Roghmann, 1975a: 127-136). A careful study by Davis (1975a, 1975b) revealed that elderly, low income Blacks in the South have only one-half as many physician visits as might be expected. She also shows that Blacks, residents of the South, Midwest, and rural areas receive proportionately fewer Medicaid benefits than do others (Davis, 1975b). Health care researchers need to investigate the important social and cultural factors distinguishing these remaining underserved populations.

Within poverty groups, there may be substantial differences in physician utilization by income and condition. Medicaid recipients, in contrast to other low income groups, have been found to use more than an expected number of physician services for nonserious conditions (Richardson, 1971; Rabin and Schach, 1975). These relatively high levels of physician utilization among the more healthy Medicaid recipients may be due to their seeking care for largely social or psychological problems and their not finding these needs met, resulting in their continued search for help (cf. Mechanic, 1976:9). Thus, it would be unwise and unfortunate if health care researchers were to turn their attention away from the critically important problems associated with financing and income due to the masking of differences by gross income group statistics.

Even with relatively equal physician utilization by income group, costs of health care may remain important for certain low income persons in their choice of medical care providers (Stratman, 1975: 547). Financial considerations may lead low income people to choose certain sources of care. However, without these income constraints, they may choose different providers whom they perceive to give better quality services. Elesh and Lefcowitz (1977) suggest that one effect of increased income gained by participants in a negative income tax experiment was that participants decided to shift their source of care from public to private providers. Analyses of volume of physician utilization alone would miss

this important role of financial considerations in the social
selection of persons into various care sources.

Indices of Access to Care

As noted above, the convergence of health care utilization rates in different income groups has led to a concern
that equality in volume of usage not be misinterpreted as an
indication of equal access to medical care. Documented
higher morbidity rates in lower income groups should imply
that they would receive more health care services than other
income groups were they achieving equality of care in relation to their need (Berkanovic and Reeder, 1974). Access to
care, it is argued, must be assessed in relation to levels of
morbidity in any group (Donabedian, 1972; Freeborn and
Greenlick, 1973).

As a response to these concerns, attempts have been
made to construct indices of access to medical care which incorporate both volume of utilization and level of morbidity
into one measure. As I feel these present problems could
lead researchers into unproductive areas, it may be useful to
review two such attempts. Aday (1975) suggests an index of
access which consists of a volume of utilization adjusted by
a measure of morbidity, i.e., the number of physician visits
divided by the number of bed or restricted activity days.
Taylor et al. (1975) suggest an index of access which relies
on expert judgments of need for medical care. A panel of
physicians rated a series of symptoms for the need they
presented for physician care. The index of access consists
of the difference between the number of symptoms reported by
an individual for which a physician visit was made and the
number of reported symptoms by this individual that the expert panel of physicians indicated should have resulted in
a physician visit.

Both of these indices are limited to the extent to
which morbidity can be adequately assessed in a survey interview situation. Using the conceptual frameworks presented,
each index can be improved through incorporation of succes-
sively more elaborate and accurate assessments of morbidity
in the population. Even then, however, such measures will
continue to ignore the relationships between perceived morbidity and sociocultural factors which have already been documented.

A major problem of the Taylor et al. index is that it
harbors the notion that there is a "proper" level of care.
As discussed earlier, medical care competes for resources
with other goods and services supplied to a society. There

is no "medical-scientific" way to determine precisely what is
needed care and what is not. This clearly depends on the
particular societal values and resources in which a medical
care system exists and morbidity occurs. For instance, what
is "proper" care as assessed by experts as appropriate for
an urban area in the United States, and as incorporated in
the Taylor et al. index, may not be "proper" care in a rural
area where physician resources are much scarcer. In other
drastically different situations, such as a rural village in
Africa in which no physician services exist, proper care is
again a rather different thing. It would be unfortunate if
assumptions hidden in this measure of access to care were to
lead researchers away from the useful insight that "proper"
care is a socially relative concept.

A second possible problem is that these indices incorporate morbidity measures in a complex variable and thus inhibit our ability to examine how morbidity relates to and
interacts with other possible influences on medical care utilization. For instance, it is important for us to learn
about the relationship between various aspects of morbidity,
such as disability-days and perceived symptoms, as these relate to social and cultural factors involved in assessment
and experience of symptoms. This is difficult to do if one
incorporates into a dependent variable what would be an independent variable for those analyses. Thus these indices
may have an inhibiting effect on our ability to understand
some complex social and cultural utilization phenomena, to
the extent that they become popularized and to the extent
that effort is put into their continual refinement rather
than into understanding how their components are related to
each other and to other social and cultural factors.

Subcultural and Ethnic Influences

Several early and remarkable studies focused on subcultural and ethnic differences in health orientations and utilization (Clark, 1959; Saunders, 1954; Zborowski, 1952).
The predominant theoretical orientation of these early works,
best expressed in Suchman's (1965, 1966) work, attributed
lower utilization among ethnic groups not yet assimilated into the broader society to their "parochial" outlook on medical issues. Persons in these ethnic groups were thought to
have less knowledge of disease and scientific medicine and to
be skeptical of more mainline medical institutions (cf. Roghmann and Haggerty, 1975: 153). Close familial and subcultural ties were thought to promote these attitudes and inhibit
medical care utilization.

While these theoretical perspectives seem to elucidate

patterns found among immigrant Irish and Italian groups as
well as Mexican-Americans and others, recent attempts at re-
plicating these theoretical propositions with regard to the
relationship between subcultural identity and use of services
have had little success (Roghmann and Haggerty, 1975). In a
study of Mormons in Salt Lake City, Geertsen et al. (1975)
found that persons better integrated into their families had
higher rates of physician utilization, the opposite of that
suggested by earlier understandings such as those proposed
by Suchman. Geertsen et al. (1975) feel that Suchman studied
more traditional ethnic groups where ethnic and family ties
promoted the anti-scientific values of these subcultures.
They feel that the Mormons studied in Salt Lake City generally held positive values towards more modern scientific medicine and that the family and cultural closeness reinforced
these values which led to higher physician use. More recent
findings such as these have alerted researchers to the fact
that subcultural and family interaction patterns are only
vehicles by which health behaviors and orientations are con-
veyed. The relationship between individuals and a variety
of subcultural groups and social movements may best be understood within this framework.

A wide variety of subcultural groups now or in the
recent past have affected health behaviors and attitudes, including the recent countercultural youth movement, the Wom-
en's Movement, Christian Science and other religious groups
with particular interest in health matters (e.g., Scientolo-
gy), as well as subcultural groups such as Mexican-Americans,
Puerto Rican migrants, and Eskimos. Each of these groups
has a different effect on certain regional populations and
groups distinct in characteristics by sex, age, and so forth.
Some such movements may have locally powerful influences by
region, last only a decade or so, and have lingering effects
on the health care system. It is difficult to fully understand a person's utilization practices without knowing his
or her integration into these subcultural groups. Especially
in this era of population sampling and efforts to have broadly representative populations, these particular distinctions
tend to be lost.

Lay Referral and Familial Interaction

Freidson (1961) observed that, before seeking professional care, individuals generally sought advice from family
and friends concerning what they should do when faced with
particular symptoms; and this pattern of advice seeking was
referred to as the "lay referral" system. Suchman (1965a:
119-120), in a study of persons with serious symptoms which
led to hospitalization or bed disability days, found that

74% of his respondents discussed these symptoms with someone
before seeking professional medical help, and 87% of these
discussions took place with relatives. Clearly the decision
to seek professional care is often made in a family context.
Robinson (1971) points out that these decision making situations involve considerably more than exchanges of information regarding symptom evaluation and sources of care. His
research emphasizes the importance of illness behavior as a
gift exchange or bargaining situation within the family.
Apart from purely financial considerations, persons assess
the burden that would be placed on other members of the family by their assumption of the sick role and what this might
mean in regard to authority relations within the family.
Family members may react to the potential patient's queries
by themselves assessing the relative burdens that the potential patient's seeking medical care might place on each family member and the likely consequences of resultant changes
in family structure and responsibilities. Family members'
advice, which is probably a major factor in utilization decisions, would likely follow in part from assessment of these
issues. These complexities are clearly insufficiently understood or researched. Considerable current reliance on cross-
sectional survey research methodology and focus on individual
decision making models of health care utilization have led
many researchers to ignore this potentially fruitful area.

Knowledge of Illness and Disease

Knowledge about illness and disease was seen by Suchman
(1965b) as possibly explaining why certain ethnic groups
used few medical services. The general argument has been
that people will use more medical services the more they
know of disease and illness. However, most studies have either found knowledge of illness and disease unrelated to use
of physician services or have found it related at only a
very minimal level (Roghmann, 1975a; Andersen, 1968;
Geertsen et al., 1975; also see McKinlay, 1972: 124-125).
While individuals may not use physician services because
they lack knowledge of disease or illness, they may also
learn of various conditions through contact with physicians,
or they may seek physician services in part because they do
not understand their condition. Uncertainty concerning
symptoms and unfamiliarity with them are thought to be important reasons for seeking medical care (Mechanic, 1968). Fear
of a disease may also lead a person to become more knowledge-
able about it; people have been found to know more about
those diseases of which they were fearful (Levine, 1962).
"Medical students' disease" is an extreme case of the opposite situation, where medical students, having learned of
various diseases, begin to fear they have these diseases and

associated symptoms and to attribute illness significance to
a variety of their bodily states which previously went unat-
tended (Mechanic, 1972a). Thus, the role of knowledge about
illness and disease in the use of acute care physician services may be more complex than can be readily understood
through research simply focusing on physician utilization as
related to knowledge of illness. Introduction of other variables such as level of fear and past experience with medical
conditions may help clarify this relationship.

Knowledge of illness and disease has been linked to
socioeconomic status. For instance, Samora et al. (1962) and
Koos (1954) find knowledge of disease conditions inversely
related to indicators of socioeconomic status. Thus, knowledge is a variable which has some potential for helping us
understand the relationship between utilization patterns and
various social and cultural statuses.

Beliefs, Attitudes and Utilization

Attitudes and beliefs concerning medical care providers
and institutions have been found useful in understanding preventive health care (Rosenstock, 1966). Suchman (1965b)
felt that lower levels of health care utilization were found
in certain ethnic groups because these groups tended to be
more skeptical of the benefits of modern medical care. Considerable effort has been made specifically to establish the
link between attitudes and beliefs about medical services
and physician utilization for acute care.

Skepticism of Medical Care

Research has focused on skepticism of medical care,
although these attitudes may be a part of a broader alienation or disaffection with societal institutions (Morris et
al., 1966). Skepticism of medical care has been measured in
a variety of ways, but it usually focuses on attitudinal
questions of potential medical care consumers as to whether
they like or dislike, trust or distrust, believe or do not
believe in the adequacy of medical services, and so forth.
Results from the International Collaborative Study of Medical
Care Utilization are reported by Bice et al. (1972) showing that skepticism of medical care is inversely related to
rates of physician visits in 11 of 12 areas studied, and
these data are used to suggest that the relationship may be
"universal". It is not possible, from the results presented,
to assess the magnitude of the relationships from this cross-
national study. A variety of other reasonably recent studies, of admittedly variable quality, have been unable to
show a relationship between skepticism of medical care and

utilization of physician services. Those studies that do
demonstrate relationships report minor to trivial associations (Hershey et al., 1975; Roghmann, 1975a; Andersen,
1968; Geertsen et al., 1975; Gaspard and Hopkins, 1967).

Beliefs about medical services may have been found generally unrelated to utilization of these services for several reasons. In developing countries that lack even minimal-
ly adequate service delivery systems and where existing services are for financial reasons inaccessible to large por-
tions of the population, it is unreasonable to believe that
attitudes and beliefs would be important relative to other
access variables (Teller, 1973). In the United States and
other Northern European countries, beliefs may be found to
have little effect on utilization because of a lack of variation in these beliefs, as suggested by the generally high
level of satisfaction reported with physician services (Ware,
1976). Finally, decisions concerning acute medical care may
simply not involve the general types of health beliefs and
attitudes that are being examined in the research cited
above. Robinson (1971) argues from his study of how people
"become ill" that individuals do not act on general beliefs
and attitudes when considering physician utilization, but
rather that their behavior is more determined by the immediate situations and concerns with which they are faced in
their personal and family lives. Similarly, Roghmann and
Haggerty (1975: 152-153) argue that health care utilization
for acute medical problems is highly impulsive and situational and is not imbedded in long-term planning strategies,
such as apparently exist in the area of preventive care
(Becker et al., 1977: 29-30). Thus health beliefs and attitudes of a general nature may not be critically important to
individuals as they make decisions about physician utilization for acute medical problems.

Past research and theorizing does suggest several possible areas for fruitful research. For instance, Anderson and
Sheatsley (1967: 45) report that 4% of their survey respondents reported delaying care because of dislike or distrust of
physicians, or feelings that physician services could not
help their problem. Relationships between skepticism of
medical care and medical care utilization could consistently
appear low or nonexistent due to the fact that this is a
major concern of such a small percentage of the total population. Skepticism of medical care may be a critical issue
and a determining factor in utilization decisions for certain
people highly alienated from our medical institutions. Future research might focus on this most disaffected group.
Attitudes toward medical care may also be important when persons are faced with diseases creating great fear, such as

cancer, and where such fears may interact with feelings that the medical system could not provide help for their problems (Kasl, 1974: 440). The interaction among skepticism of medical care, fear of disease, and perceived vulnerability is a promising area for investigation. While most conceptualizations of health beliefs relate them to socialization in various ethnic and subcultural groups (Zborowski, 1952; Zola, 1964; Suchman, 1965b, 1965c), very little research has been done on childhood socialization of health beliefs and behaviors (for an exception see Mechanic, 1964). Finally, increasing evidence exists that skepticism of medical care related to particular providers may result in "shopping for doctors" and choice of particular medical care facilities (Kasteler et al., 1976; Franklin and McLemore, 1970; Anderson and Bartkus, 1973). Subcultural attitudes and beliefs about medical care may also serve to divert people from general health care facilities into alternate types of care. In a study of students' use of professional help for psychological problems, students who used psychiatrists were more likely to have campus counter-cultural attitudes and to have positive views of psychiatrists, while students not sharing these attitudes were more likely to seek help from counsellors, clergymen, nonpsychiatrist physicians, and so forth (Greenley and Mechanic, 1976a). Overall rates of seeking help differed little by attitudes, but attitudes were strongly related to the source of help sought. Thus, attitudinal factors may result in a person seeking care not from a physician but through chiropractors, faith healers, curanderos, and other alternative practitioners (Saunders, 1954).

Tendency to Adopt the Sick Role

Considerable research has focused on the relationship between health care utilization and the "tendency to seek medical care" (Kirscht, 1974: 397-398; Kasl, 1974: 438). One of the earlier and more important measures of this concept was Mechanic and Volkart's (1961) measure of the "tendency to adopt the sick role". They presented individuals with certain symptoms and asked them to indicate whether they would seek physician care if they had these symptoms. Persons who responded positively that they would seek care for more of these symptoms were considered to have a higher tendency to adopt the sick role. Other researchers have used this basic strategy for assessing concepts known by a wide variety of names: "the readiness to seek medical care" (Koos, 1954); "the tendency to use services" (Bice and White, 1969); "the readiness to act" (Battistella, 1968); "symptom sensitivity" (Hetherington and Hopkins, 1969); and "the readiness to seek care" (Roghmann, 1975a). (Also see Hankin, 1974; Monteiro, 1973; Bice et al., 1972.) In general, persons who express a greater tendency to adopt the sick role also have been found to make greater use of physician services, although these relationships are usually small and sometimes statistically insignificant.

Measures of the tendency to adopt the sick role have been shown to be related to a variety of social and demographic characteristics such as sex, age, and socioeconomic group (Monteiro, 1973; Hetherington and Hopkins, 1969; Anderson and Bartkus, 1973). However, efforts to demonstrate that the tendency to adopt the sick role is an explanatory variable linking such social or demographic characteristics to volume of health care utilization have been disappointing (see Greenley and Mechanic, 1976a), no doubt in part due to the consistently low degree of association between tendency to adopt the sick role and measures of utilization (Roghmann, 1975a; Hankin, 1974).

A major problem with this concept is evidenced by the variety of names given these measures which are built in logically similar ways. Kasl (1974: 438) notes that measures of tendency to adopt the sick role may be seen as assessments of symptom severity. Hetherington and Hopkins (1969) saw this type of measure as indicating "symptom sensitivity"; and Kirscht (1974: 397) notes that such measures also may be seen as indicators of values placed on medical care. Indeed, interview questions designed to measure tendency to adopt the sick role include assessment of severity of symptoms, appropriateness of taking these symptoms to physicians, possible efficacy of physician's services in dealing with these symptoms, and competing values and obligations affecting persons' assessment of whether a physician's visit would be worthwhile for any particular symptom. Thus, were refinements of this type of measure to suddenly produce substantial relationships between the concept "tendency to adopt the sick role" and utilization, these would appear to be difficult to interpret theoretically. This important concept of the sick role has been critically useful in sensitizing us to the importance of social and cultural factors in the decision to seek medical care. However, further research advances and understanding of utilization behaviors may best be served by a focus on more refined measures which essentially decompose the various aspects of the decision-making task posed by measures of tendency to adopt the sick role. This would greatly aid our attempts to build theoretical models of increasing sophistication. A measure of tendency to adopt the sick role may remain useful only as a gross composite measure of the many factors it incorporates; for instance, it may be used as a control variable in studies of physician utilization under various payment plans.

Other Psychosocial Factors in Utilization

A variety of other psychological and social concepts
and variables have been used in the study of health care utilization. None of these has been focused on to nearly the
extent that knowledge of health and disease, tendency to
adopt the sick role, or skepticism of medical care has been.
There is a general lack of information regarding these concepts, and it is therefore difficult to assess their future
utility in theoretical or empirical work in health care utilization. These psychological and psychosocial variables
are not necessarily conceptually distinct nor are there
clearly agreed upon measures for any one of them. First,
alienation has been found to be an important predictor of
preventive care. While greater alienation has been generally related to lower levels of preventive medical care, Hoppe
and Heller (1975) found that greater alienation was related
to higher levels of physician use, using a measure of alienation focusing on "powerlessness". Alienation, which is
variously measured and defined, focuses on a general disaffection with and feelings of nonparticipation in societal
institutions. It may be, as noted above, closely related to
skepticism of medical care. As alienation is commonly measured, it is similar to life stress and general psychological
distress measures, which, as we shall see below, are themselves promising concepts in our attempt to understand
health care utilization. Thus, it is difficult to interpret
even the few existing findings regarding utilization and
alienation.

Suchman (1965a) suggested that the tendency to be dependent in illness was an important psychosocial concept.
However, recent studies have not found it related to health
care utilization (Roghmann, 1975a; Geertsen et al., 1975).
A belief in lack of individual control over one's life and
especially health related concerns, often called fatalism,
has been suggested as a possible psychological variable affecting health care utilization. Research on fatalism,
however, has not been encouraging; Hershey et al. (1975),
for instance, did not find fatalism related to health care
utilization.

Specific fears of illness and disease have been noted
as important in the avoidance of care. Anderson and Sheatsley (1967: 45) report 4% of their survey respondents studied
indicated delay in seeking care for symptomatic conditions
due to fear of a particular diagnosis or treatment. Becker
et al. (1977: 33), in a review of relevant literature, suggest that health actions are inhibited at some threshold

level of fear. Specific health related fears, possibly related to general feelings of vulnerability, may be critical variables in health care utilization in certain circumstances and for some people. Research in this area has been minimal and has produced somewhat conflicting results (Gochman, 1972; Roghmann, 1975a). Fear of disease may result in denial of illness (Antonovsky, 1972). Denial of illness may also arise out of other competing values and cultural orientations such as the Protestant ethic in our society, which may lead people to deny symptoms in order that they may continue pursuing valued vocational and other social activities. The role of competing values in denial of illness and fear of disease is an under-researched area.

Psychological Distress and Utilization

Many physicians have long suspected that persons experiencing higher levels of psychological distress use more than their share of physician services. In the past, the empirical evidence to support this proposition has long been inconclusive, due to numerous methodological difficulties. However, a number of relatively recent studies with substantially improved methodology lead us to conclude with increasing assurance that persons experiencing higher levels of psychological distress do have generally higher rates of physician utilization (Shepherd et al., 1966; Tessler et al., 1976; Roghmann and Haggerty, 1975; Hankin, 1974; Cummings and Follette, 1968). These are generally prospective studies predicting physician utilization from measures of psychological distress obtained before utilization is assessed and independent of the physician's care itself. While associations between psychological distress and utilization in these studies are generally modest, in some studies they are similar in magnitude to associations between measures of morbidity and physician utilization (Tessler et al., 1976: 362-363).

Persons experiencing psychological distress are perhaps over-represented among chronically high users of medical care. In one study of the Health Insurance Plan of New York, 14% of plan members used 52% of the services (4% used almost 25% of all services used), and there appeared to be a substantial tendency for high utilizers to remain high utilizers over time (Densen et al., 1959). Kogan et al. (1975) found a similar pattern among members of the Puget Sound Group Health Cooperative and noted that high utilizers of health services tended to be persons receiving mental health care at that time.

Psychological Distress and the Etiology of Illness

One explanation for this relationship between psychological distress and patterns of utilization lies in the well-documented association between life stress and physical illness (Dohrenwend and Dohrenwend, 1974). Because persons who experience stress in their lives or are psychologically distressed have been shown to have higher levels of a wide variety of illnesses and conditions, Tessler et al. (1976) examined the relationship between physician utilization and psychological distress, statistically controlling for measures of physical morbidity, and found the relationship remained. The available data suggest that psychologically distressed persons use more physician services than would be expected even given their generally higher levels of morbidity.

Psychological Distress as a Trigger for Utilization

Another set of explanations focuses on psychological distress as a possible trigger to health care utilization. First, psychological distress may trigger physician utilization by enhancing sensitivity to symptomatic conditions or causing persons to assess symptoms as more serious or threatening. Zola (1964) hypothesized that "interpersonal crises" may call attention to symptoms and thus lead to more physician utilization. Also, psychological distress may distort perceptions of symptoms and conditions, amplifying their seriousness to an abnormal degree (Mechanic, 1968). Persons with neurotic conditions may tend to focus excessively on their symptoms or worry about them to an unusual degree, leading them possibly to over-report symptoms in medical care surveys (Mechanic and Newton, 1965). Therefore, distressed individuals have been observed to report themselves in worse health than nondistressed individuals, controlling for other measures of health status (Tessler and Mechanic, 1978). A study of hysterical contagion among women employees of a Southern mill found that employees reporting themselves ill were more often those who had personal problems they could not admit to or deal with (Kerckhoff and Back, 1968). One interpretation of this phenomenon suggests that these employees were in stressful situations that may have made them more sensitive to transient, minor, or preexisting conditions which they equated with symptoms of the presumed "illness".

Second, psychological distress may increase physician utilization by reducing individuals' coping abilities to the point where they feel need for professional help (Roghmann and Haggerty, 1975: 142 ff). Acute care is often sought in the context of uncertainty concerning symptoms and conditions, and psychological distress may make individuals less able to cope with uncertainty (cf. Becker et al., 1977: 29-30). Psychological distress may reduce one's level of tolerance to symptomatic conditions (Mechanic, 1968), or may make people feel more vulnerable to illness.

Third, psychological distress may be related to utilization due to relationships of psychological distress to skepticism of medical care or feelings of personal control. Psychological distress may also be related to tendency to adopt the sick role in complex ways; Mechanic and Volkart (1961) report that stress may trigger help seeking among those with a high tendency to adopt the sick role. Tessler et al. (1976), however, examined the relationship between psychological distress and physician utilization, controlling for propensity to seek medical care, skepticism of medical care, and perceived personal control. They found that there was no evidence that psychologically distressed persons use more physician services due to these attitudes or orientations.

Psychological Distress and the Search for Services

A third set of explanations for the relationship between psychological distress and physician utilization suggests that psychologically distressed persons overtly or covertly take their personal social and psychological problems to physicians in search of help. Balint (1957) argued that many persons bringing somatic complaints to physicians were merely disguising their search for help with personal problems. The argument is that persons bring physical symptoms to physicians as "entry tickets" into physician care for the obscured purpose of dealing with their unrevealed personal problems or "latent needs" (Tessler et al., 1976). For various reasons, people may have difficulty expressing emotional problems, and they may feel more comfortable revealing physical complaints instead. Zborowski (1952) described the socialization of children of "old American" families, noting that they were taught to take illness "like a man" and "not cry". He suggests that this would not necessarily discourage the use of physicians as much as make for the presentation of physical rather than emotional complaints. Bart (1968) compared women coming to a neurology clinic, and who were subsequently referred to a psychiatry service, to women who sought care directly from the psychiatry service. She felt that the women referred from the neurology to the psychiatry service were expressing psychological problems in physical terms. In the study of hysterical contagion in the Southern mill discussed above, it is implied that the women adopted a view of themselves as physically ill in part because they could not face and deal with personal problems in an open manner (Kerckhoff and Back, 1968). These and other data suggest that individuals who are psychologically distressed take personal problems to physicians in search of relief of these problems even if they do not realize that this may be their underlying purpose or need.

Psychologically distressed individuals may also have higher rates of physician utilization because they recognize their personal problems and consciously choose to take them to physicians for discussion and advice. Gurin et al. (1960), for instance, found that 30% of persons reporting personal problems and subsequently seeking help with them initially took their problems to nonpsychiatrist physicians. Greenley and Mechanic (1976b: 187) found that, in a three-month period, while 2% of their college student respondents took personal problems for discussion to psychiatrists or other mental health professionals, 2% took their problems to a University Counseling Service, and 3% sought help from religious counselors, the largest reported source of care was physicians; 6% took their personal problems to nonpsychiatrist physicians (also see Satin, 1973). The extent to which patients see themselves as taking personal and psychological problems to physicians should not be underestimated. However, patients may acknowledge in surveys that they take personal problems to physicians but do not overtly present their problems to the physicians themselves; such patients may present somatic complaints to physicians in order to legitimize their visit. In sum, available data suggest that psychologically distressed individuals use more physician services because they overtly or covertly take psychological or personal problems to physicians for their aid.

Physician Response to Psychological Distress

The response of physicians and medical personnel to their patients' personal and psychological problems may have an impact on the volume and pattern of utilization. This author's estimate, based on some available information, suggests that physicians prescribe psychoactive medications, mostly minor tranquilizers, to patients on approximately 10% of all visits (NCHS, 1976: 17; Josephson and Carroll, 1974). To the extent that such prescriptions are temporary responses to symptomatic complaints rather than attempts to deal with social or psychological problems, physicians may be responding in a way that ends up producing repeat visits for symptomatic relief of ongoing problems. To the extent that physicians may interpret requests for help with personal problems, whether or not presented as physical symptoms, as evidence of physical disorders, they may inadvertently treat people for physical illnesses in unnecessary and potentially costly ways (Bart, 1968). In these ways, physician responses to patient requests for help with personal and psychological problems may affect utilization rates.

Physician responses may also affect the selection of care by patients. Kasteler et al. (1976) found "doctor shopping" more prevalent among those scoring high on a hypochondriasis scale, and Tessler et al. (1976) found that, among their study sample of members in a prepaid medical care plan, out-of-plan usage was greater for those expressing more psychological distress. Patient uncertainty, worry, and excessive sensitivity to symptoms, or insufficiently appropriate physician responses may lead patients to seek a variety of alternative sources of care such as chiropractic, faith healing, and so forth.

Measures of psychological distress used in studies in this area ask about symptoms and conditions which may be produced by transient life stresses or by more neurotic personality patterns. Therefore, it is not possible to determine whether one or both of these sources of psychological distress may be more responsible for the existing evidence of greater physician utilization among those expressing this distress. Careful work using intensive interviews and health diaries by Robinson (1971) and Roghmann and Haggerty (1975) suggests to me that transient stress and associated psychological distress may be the more important factor in health care utilization decisions. They emphasize the immediate and somewhat impulsive nature of health care utilization decisions and the extent to which they are conditioned on particular situational factors in a person's vocational and family life.

Conclusion

This paper has attempted to review selected major issues concerning social and psychological factors in health care utilization. While our focus has been on ambulatory utilization of physician services for acute care problems, many of the issues raised and conclusions drawn are applicable to other areas in the study of medical care utilization. An attempt has been made to critically evaluate past research and theory, with a particular focus on recent work.

Health care utilization behavior is affected by patients' sociopsychological characteristics as those influence patient reactions to and interactions with health care institutions. This critical area, which is beyond the scope of this paper, needs careful review and consideration (McKinlay, 1972).

While no separate attempt was made to evaluate methodological procedures, several observations were made. The need to focus on more narrowly defined and unique types of utilization behavior was noted, and the utility of attempting to understand or explain aggregated utilization measures was questioned. The need for prospective studies of utilization behavior was noted; gathering attitudinal and psychological information to predict previous utilization should clearly be avoided. Because existing data indicate that various sociopsychological factors are related to patterns of reporting of health care utilization (NCHSR, 1975), survey researchers should not attempt to gather from patients both measures of utilization and measures of sociopsychological variables used to predict utilization. Whenever possible, measures of health care utilization should be obtained separately from provider records. The utility of using intensive case studies and health diaries was noted. Recent attempts to devise indices of access to care which incorporate both measures of morbidity and indicators of utilization of health care were seen as generally unwise, because these indices would inhibit our ability to understand the relationships among utilization behaviors, morbidity, and sociopsychological factors.

Limited use should be made of currently devised measures of "tendency to adopt a sick role". These measures should be decomposed into their component concepts in order to make the data more theoretically interpretable.

A wide variety of promising questions was noted, only a few of which will be reviewed here. How is psychological distress related to physician utilization? Does psychological distress cause individuals to be more sensitive to symptoms, to need social support which they seek from physicians, or, does psychological distress operate in some other way to influence physician utilization? What are the utilization consequences of how physicians deal with patients who present overt or latent social or personal problems? What makes people aware of abnormal bodily states and attribute illness significance to them? What attitudes and beliefs, apart from those directly related to medical care, reduce utilization through provision of conflicting motivations?

Particular attention should be paid to exploration of theoretical "models" which focus on immediate situational and contextual factors around which utilization decisions are made. Theories which incorporate a view of physician utilization as more impulsive and irrational than usually considered may need to be developed.

It is important that these critiques and suggestions not obscure the tremendous advances that have been made by behavioral scientists in their attempts to understand social-cultural and psychological aspects of medical care utilization. Continued productive work on these issues requires that we adopt new concepts and new methods in order to build on the firm base of theory and research in this area which now exists.

References

Aday, LuAnn and Robert Eichhorn. The Utilization of Health Services: Ideas and Correlates. Washington: National Center for Health Services Research and Development. U.S. Department of HEW Publication No. (HSM) 73-3003, 1972.

Aday, LuAnn. "Economic and Noneconomic Barriers to the Use of Needed Medical Services." Medical Care XIII, 6 (June, 1975): 447-456.

Andersen, Ronald. A Behavioral Model of Families' Use of Health Services. Center for Health Administration Studies, Research Series No. 25. Chicago: University of Chicago, 1968.

Andersen, Ronald, Odin W. Anderson, and Bjorn Smedby. "Perception of and Response to Symptoms in Sweden and the United States." Medical Care VI, (January-February, 1968): 18-30.

Anderson, James G. and David E. Bartkus. "Choice of Medical Care: A Behavioral Model of Health and Illness Behavior." Journal of Health and Social Behavior 14 (December, 1973): 348-362.

Anderson, Odin W. and Paul B. Sheatsley. Hospital Use: A Survey of Patient and Physician Decisions. Center for Health Administration Studies, Research Series No. 24. Chicago: University of Chicago, 1967.

Anderson, Odin W. and Ronald M. Andersen. "Patterns of Use of Health Services." Pp. 386-406 in H. Freeman, S. Levine, and L. Reeder, eds., Handbook of Medical Sociology. Englewood Cliffs, N.J.: Prentice-Hall, 1972.

Antonovsky, Aaron. "A Model to Explain Visits to the Doctor:
    With Specific Reference to the Case of Israel." Journal
    of Health and Social Behavior 13, 4 (December, 1972):
    446-454.

Balint, Michael. The Doctor, His Patient, and the Illness.
    New York: International Universities Press, 1957.

Bart, Pauline B. "Social Structure and Vocabularies of Dis-
    comfort: What Happened to Female Hysteria?" Journal
    of Health and Social Behavior 9, 3 (September, 1968):
    188-193.

Battistella, R. "Limitations in Use of the Concept of Psy-
    chological Readiness to Initiate Health Care." Medical
    Care 6 (July-August, 1968): 308-319.

Becker, Howard S. Outsiders: Studies in the Sociology of
    Deviance. New York: Free Press, 1963.

Becker, Marshall H., Don P. Haefner, Stanislav V. Kasl, John
    P. Kirscht, Lois A. Maiman, and Irwin M. Rosenstock.
    "Selected Psychosocial Models and Correlates of Indivi-
    dual Health-Related Behaviors." Medical Care XV, 5,
    supplement (May, 1977): 27-46.

Berkanovic, Emil and Leo G. Reeder. "Can Money Buy the Ap-
    propiate Use of Services? Some Notes on the Meaning
    of Utilization Data." Journal of Health and Social
    Behavior 15, 2 (June, 1974): 93-99.

Bice, Thomas and Kerr L. White. "Factors Related to the Use
    of Health Services: An International Comparative Study."
    Medical Care VII, 2 (March-April, 1969): 124-133.

Bice, Thomas W. and Kerr L. White. "Cross-National Compara-
    tive Research on the Utilization of Medical Services."
    Medical Care IX, 3 (May-June, 1971):253-270.

Bice, Thomas W., Robert L. Eichorn, and Peter O. Fox. "So-
    cioeconomic Status and Use of Physician Services: A
    Reconsideration." Medical Care X, 3 (May-June, 1972):
    261-271.

Bice, Thomas W., David L. Rabin, Barbara H. Starfield, and
    Kerr L. White. "Economic Class and Use of Physician
    Services." Medical Care XI, 4 (July-August, 1973):
    287-296.

Clark, Margaret. Health in the Mexican-American Culture. Berkeley: University of California Press, 1959.

Cooper, Barbara S. "National Health Expenditures, Fiscal Years 1929-1969 and Calendar Years 1929-1968." Research and Statistics, Note 18, Social Security Administration, November 2, 1969.

Cummings, Nicholas A. and William T. Follette. "Psychiatric Service and Medical Utilization in a Prepaid Health Plan Setting. Part II." Medical Care VI (January-February, 1968): 31-41.

Davis, Karen. "Equal Treatment and Unequal Benefits: The Medicare Program." Milbank Memorial Fund Quarterly (Health and Society), 53 (Fall, 1975a): 449-488.

Davis, Karen. National Health Insurance: Benefits, Costs, and Consequences. Washington, D.C.: The Brookings Institution, 1975b.

Densen, Paul, Sam Shapiro, and Marilyn Einhorn. "Concerning High and Low Utilization of Service in a Medical Care Plan and the Persistence of Utilization Levels Over a Three Year Period." Milbank Memorial Fund Quarterly (Health and Society), 37 (July, 1959): 217-250.

Dohrenwend, Barbara Snell and Bruce P. Dohrenwend. Stressful Life Events: Their Nature and Effects. New York: Wiley and Sons, 1974.

Donabedian, Avedis. "Models for Organizing Delivery of Personal Health Service." Milbank Memorial Fund Quarterly (Health and Society), 50 (October, 1972): 103-154.

Elesh, David and M. Jack Lefcowitz. "The Effects of the New Jersey-Pennsylvania Negative Income Tax Experiment on Health and Health Care Utilization." Journal of Health and Social Behavior 18, 4 (December, 1977): 391-405.

Fabrega, Horacio. "Toward a Model of Illness Behavior." Medical Care XI, 6 (November-December, 1973): 470-484.

Falk, Isadore S., Margaret C. Klein, and Nathan Sinai. The Incidence of Illness and the Receipt and Costs of Medical Care Among Representative Families: Experiences in Twenty Consecutive Months During 1928-31. Committee on the Cost of Medical Care Report, No. 26. Chicago:

University of Chicago Press, 1933.

Fink, Raymond. "The Measurement of Medical Care Utiliza-
    tion." Pp. 5-32 in M.R. Greenlick, ed., Conceptual
    Issues in the Analysis of Medical Care Utilization
    Behavior. U.S. Department of HEW: Public Health Ser-
    vice, 1969.

Franklin, Billy Joe and S. Dale McLemore. "Factors Affect-
    ing the Choice of Medical Care Among University Stu-
    dents." Journal of Health and Social Behavior 11, 4
    (December, 1970): 311-319.

Freeborn, Donald K. and Merwyn R. Greenlick. "Evaluation of
    the Performance of Ambulatory Care Systems: Research
    Requirements and Opportunities." Medical Care XI,
    (March-April, 1973, Supplement): 68-75.

Freidson, Eliot. Patients' Views of Medical Practice. New
    York: Russell Sage Foundation, 1961.

Galvin, Michael E. and Margaret Fan. "The Utilization of
    Physicians' Services in Los Angeles County, 1973."
    Journal of Health and Social Behavior 16, 1 (March,
    1975): 74-94.

Gaspard, Nancy J. and Carl E. Hopkins. "Determinants of Use
    of Ambulatory Medical Services by an Aged Population."
    Inquiry (A Review of Current Research in Hospital and
    Medical Economics), 4 (March, 1967): 28-36.

Geertsen, Reed, Melville R. Klauber, Mark Rindflesh, Robert
    L. Kane, and Robert Gray. "A Re-examination of Such-
    man's Views on Social Factors in Health Care Utiliza-
    tion." Journal of Health and Social Behavior 16, 2
    (June, 1975): 226-237.

Gochman, David S. "The Organizing Role of Motivation in
    Health Beliefs and Intentions." Journal of Health and
    Social Behavior 13, 3 (September, 1972): 285-293.

Greenley, James R. and David Mechanic. "Social Selection in
    Seeking Help for Psychological Problems." Journal of
    Health and Social Behavior 17, 3 (September, 1976a):
    249-262.

Greenley, James R. and David Mechanic. "Patterns of Seeking
    Care for Psychological Problems." Pp. 177-196 in D.
    Mechanic, ed., The Growth of Bureaucratic Medicine.
    New York: John Wiley & Sons, 1976b.

Greenlick, Merwyn R., Arnold V. Hurtado, Clyde R. Pope, Ernest W. Saward, and Samuel S. Yoshioka. "Determinants of Medical Care Utilization." Health Services Research 3 (Winter, 1968): 296-315.

Guillozet, Noel. "Community Mental Health--New Approaches for Rural Areas Using Psychiatric Social Workers." Medical Care XIII, 1 (January, 1975): 59-67.

Gurin, Gerald, Joseph Veroff, and Sheila Feld. Americans View the Mental Health. New York: Basic Books, 1960.

Guttmacher, Sally and Jack Elinson. "Ethno-Religious Variation in Perceptions of Illness." Social Science and Medicine 5 (April, 1971): 117-125.

Hammond, E. Cuyler. "Some Preliminary Findings on Physical Complaints from a Prospective Study of 1,064,004 Men and Women." American Journal of Public Health 54, 1 (January, 1964): 11-23.

Hankin, Janet R. Psychological Distress and the Use of Medical Services. Unpublished Ph.D. Dissertation, University of Wisconsin-Madison, 1974.

Hershey, John C., Harold S. Luft, and Joan M. Gianaris. "Making Sense Out of Utilization Data." Medical Care XIII, 10 (October, 1975): 838-854.

Hetherington, Robert W. and Carl E. Hopkins. "Symptom Sensitivity: Its Social and Cultural Correlates." Health Services Research 4 (Spring, 1969): 63-75.

Hoppe, Sue Keir and Peter L. Heller. "Alienation, Familism and the Utilization of Health Services by Mexican-Americans." Journal of Health and Social Behavior 16, 3 (September, 1975): 304-314.

Hulka, Barbara S., Lawrence Kupper, and John C. Cassel. "Determinants of Physician Utilization." Medical Care X (July-August, 1972): 300-309.

Hyman, Martin D. "Some Links Between Socioeconomic Status and Untreated Illness." Social Science and Medicine 4 (November, 1970): 387-399.

Josephson, Eric and Eleanor E. Carroll. Drug Use: Epidemiological and Sociological Approaches. Washington: Hemisphere Publishing Company, 1974.

Kadushin, Charles. "Individual Decisions to Undertake Psychotherapy." Administrative Science Quarterly 3 (December, 1958-1959): 379-411.

Kalimo, Esko, Robert Kohn, and Branko Bedenic. "Interrelationships in the Use of Selected Health Services: A Cross-National Study." Medical Care X (March-April, 1972): 95-108.

Kasl, Stanislav V. "The Health Belief Model and Behavior Related to Chronic Illness." Health Education Monographs 2, 4 (Winter, 1974): 433-454.

Kasl, Stanislav V. and S. Cobb. "Health Behavior, Illness Behavior, and Sick Role Behavior. I. Health and Illness Behavior." Archives of Environmental Health 12 (February, 1966): 246-266.

Kasteler, Josephine, Robert L. Kane, Donna M. Olsen, and Constance Thetford. "Issues Underlying Prevalence of 'Doctor-Shopping' Behavior." Journal of Health and Social Behavior 17, 4 (December, 1976): 328-339.

Kerckhoff, Alan C. and Kurt W. Back. The June Bug: A Study of Hysterical Contagion. New York: Appleton-Century-Croft, 1968.

Kirscht, John P. "The Health Belief Model and Illness Behavior." Health Education Monographs 2, 4 (Winter, 1974): 387-408.

Kogan, William S., Donovan J. Thompson, Jack R. Brown, and Harold F. Newman. "Impact of Integration of Mental Health Service and Comprehensive Medical Care." Medical Care XIII, 11 (November, 1975): 934-942.

Koos, Earl. The Health of Regionville: What the People Thought and Did About It. New York: Columbia University Press, 1954.

Levine, Gene N. "Anxiety about Illness: Psychological and Social Bases." Journal of Health and Human Behavior 3, 1 (Spring, 1962): 30-34.

Lewis, Charles E., Rashi Fein, and David Mechanic. A Right to Health. New York: John Wiley, 1976.

McKinlay, John B. "Some Approaches and Problems in the Study of the Use of Services - An Overview." Journal of Health and Social Behavior 13, 2 (June, 1972): 115-152.

McKinlay, John B. and Diana B. Dutton. "Social-Psychological Factors Affecting Health Service Utilization." Pp. 251-303 in S. Mushkin, ed., Consumer Incentives for Health Care. New York: Prodist, 1974.

Mechanic, David. "The Concept of Illness Behavior." Journal of Chronic Diseases 15 (February, 1962): 189-194.

Mechanic, David. "Religion, Religiosity, and Illness Behavior: The Special Case of the Jews." Human Organization 22, 3 (Fall, 1963): 202-208.

Mechanic, David. "The Influence of Mothers on Their Children's Health Attitudes and Behavior." Pediatrics 33 (March, 1964): 444-453.

Mechanic, David. Medical Sociology: A Selective View. New York: The Free Press, 1968.

Mechanic, David. "Illness and Cure." Pp. 191-214 in J. Kosa, A. Antonovsky, and I. Zola, eds., Poverty and Health (1st edition). Cambridge: Harvard University Press, 1969.

Mechanic, David. "Social Psychologic Factors Affecting the Presentation of Bodily Complaints." New England Journal of Medicine 286 (May 25, 1972a): 1132-1139.

Mechanic, David. Public Expectations and Health Care. New York: Wiley-Interscience, 1972b.

Mechanic, David. "The Problems of Access to Medical Care." Pp. 3-13 in Charles E. Lewis, R. Fein, and David Mechanic, eds., A Right to Health. New York: Wiley & Sons, 1976.

Mechanic, David and M. Newton. "Some Problems in the Analysis of Morbidity Data." Journal of Chronic Diseases 18 (June, 1965): 569-580.

Mechanic, David and E. Volkart. "Stress, Illness Behavior and the Sick Role." American Sociological Review 26, 1 (February, 1961): 51-58.

Monteiro, Lois A. "Expense is No Object...: Income and Physician Visits Reconsidered." Journal of Health and Social Behavior 14, 2 (June, 1973): 99-115.

Morris, Naomi, Martha Hatch, and Sidney Chipman. "Alienation as a Deterrent to Well-Child Supervision." American Journal of Public Health 56 (November, 1966): 1874-
1882.

National Center for Health Service Research. Advances in
Health Survey Research Methods. Washington, D.C.: U.S.
Department of HEW. Publication No. (HRA): 77-3154,
1975.

National Center for Health Statistics. Health Characteristics of Low Income Persons. Series 10, No. (HSM):
73-1500, July, 1972.

National Center for Health Statistics. The Nation's Use of
Health Resources: 1976 Edition. U.S. Department of
HEW. Publication No. (HRA): 77-1240, 1976.

Newhouse, Joseph P., Charles E. Phelps, and William B.
Schwartz. "Policy Options and the Impact of National
Health Insurance." New England Journal of Medicine 290
(June 13, 1974): 1345-1359.

Quesada, Gustavo M. and Peter L. Heller. "Sociocultural
Barriers to Medical Care among Mexican Americans in
Texas." Medical Care XV, 5, Supplement (May, 1977):
93-101.

Rabin, David L. and Elisabeth Schach. "Medicaid, Morbidity,
and Physician Use." Medical Care XIII, 1 (January,
1975): 68-78.

Restuccia, Joseph D. and Don C. Holloway. "Barriers to Appropriate Utilization of an Acute Facility." Medical
Care XIV, 7 (July, 1976): 559-573.

Richardson, William C. Ambulatory Use of Physician's Ser-
vices in Response to Illness Episodes in a Low Income
Neighborhood. Research Series 29, Center for Health
Administration Studies. Chicago: University of Chicago
Press, 1971.

Robinson, David. The Process of Becoming Ill. London:
Routledge and Kegan Paul, 1971.

Roemer, Milton I., Carl E. Hopkins, Lockwood Carr, and
Foline Gartside. "Copayments for Ambulatory Care:
Penny-wise and Pound-foolish." Medical Care XIII, 6
(June, 1975): 457-466.

Roghmann, Klaus J. "Models of Health and Illness Behavior: A. Available Models." Pp. 119-141 in R. Haggerty, K. Roghmann, and I. Pless, eds., Child Health and the Community. New York: Wiley-Interscience, 1975a.

Roghmann, Klaus J. "The Utilization of Health Service." Pp. 169-196 in R. Haggerty, K. Roghmann, and I. Pless, eds., Child Health and the Community. New York: Wiley-Interscience, 1975b.

Roghmann, Klaus J. and Robert J. Haggerty. "The Stress Model for Illness Behavior." Pp. 142-156 in R. Haggerty, K. Roghmann, and I. Pless, eds., Child Health and the Community. New York: Wiley-Interscience, 1975.

Rosenstock, Irwin M. "Why People Use Health Services." Milbank Memorial Fund Quarterly (Health and Society) 44, Part II, 3 (July, 1966): 94-124.

Salber, Eva J., Sandra B. Greene, Jacob J. Feldman, and Georgia Hunter. "Access to Health Care in a Southern Rural Community." Medical Care XIV, 12 (December, 1976): 971-986.

Samora, Julian, Lyla Saunders, and Richard F. Larson. "Knowledge about Specific Diseases in Four Selected Samples." Journal of Health and Human Behavior 3, 3 (Fall, 1962): 176-185.

Satin, David George. "'Help': The Hospital Emergency Unit Patient and His Presenting Picture." Medical Care XI, 4 (July-August, 1973): 328-337.

Saunders, Lyle. Cultural Differences and Medical Care. New York: Russell Sage Foundation, 1954.

Scheff, Thomas J. Being Mentally Ill: A Sociological Theory. Chicago: Aldine, 1966.

Shepherd, Michael, Brian Cooper, Alexander C. Brown, and Graham Kalton. Psychiatric Illness in General Practice. London: Oxford University Press, 1966.

Shuval, Judith T. Social Functions of Medical Practice. San Francisco: John Wiley, 1970.

Stratmann, William C. "A Study of Consumer Attitudes about Health Care: The Delivery of Ambulatory Services." Medical Care XIII, 7 (July, 1975): 537-548.

Suchman, Edward A. "Stages of Illness and Medical Care." Journal of Health and Human Behavior 6, 3 (Fall, 1965a): 114-128.

Suchman, Edward A. "Social Patterns of Illness and Medical Care." Journal of Health and Human Behavior 6, 1 (Spring, 1965b): 2-16.

Suchman, Edward A. "Social Factors in Medical Deprivation." American Journal of Public Health 55, 11 (November, 1965c): 1725-1733.

Suchman, Edward A. "Health Orientation and Medical Care." American Journal of Public Health 56 (January, 1966): 97-105.

Taylor, D. Garth, LuAnn Aday, and Ronald Andersen. "A Social Indicator of Access to Medical Care." Journal of Health and Social Behavior 16, 1 (March, 1975): 39-49.

Teller, Charles H. "Access to Medical Care of Migrants in a Honduran City." Journal of Health and Social Behavior 14, 3 (September, 1973): 214-225.

Tessler, Richard and David Mechanic. "Psychological Distress and Perceived Health Status." Journal of Health and Social Behavior (forthcoming), 1978.

Tessler, Richard, David Mechanic, and Margaret Dimond. "The Effect of Psychological Distress on Physician Utilization: A Prospective Study." Journal of Health and Social Behavior 17, 4 (December, 1976): 353-364.

Ware, John E., Mary K. Snyder, and W. Russell Wright. Development and Validation of Scales to Measure Patient Satisfaction with Health Care Services: Volume 1 of a Final Report. Part A: Review of Literature, Overview of Methods and Results Regarding Construction of Scales. Carbondale, Ill.: Southern Illinois School of Medicine, 1976.

Welch, Susan, John Comer, and Michael Steinman. "Some Social and Attitudinal Correlates of Health Care Among Mexican-Americans." Journal of Health and Social Behavior 14 (September, 1973): 205-213.

Zborowski, M. "Cultural Components in Response to Pain." Journal of Social Issues 8, 4 (1952):16-30.

Zola, Irving K. "Illness Behavior of the Working Class: Implications and Recommendations." Pp. 350-361 in A.B. Shostak and W. Gomberg, eds., Blue Collar World: Studies of the American Worker. Englewood Cliffs, New Jersey: Prentice Hall, 1964.

Zola, Irving K. "Culture and Symptoms: An Analysis of Patients' Presenting Complaints." American Sociological Review 31 (October, 1966): 615-630.

7. The Bearing of Social Sciences Knowledge on Medical Education and Practice

When Oliver Wendell Holmes spoke in 1860 about the state of medical therapy, he was driven to comment: "I firmly believe that if the whole materia medica, as now used, could be sunk to the bottom of the sea, it would be all the better for mankind--and all the worse for the fishes." (Holmes, 1883)

Some may still agree that Dr. Holmes' suggestion continues to have merit. But most would not. Most physicians and laymen praise the advances in medical technique of the past century, which cure diseases before fatal, relieve suffering before stoically borne, and increase the expectancy of human life. They express an appropriate fidelity and gratitude to the engines of this progress, the physical, chemical, and biological sciences; and to the temples of science in which the disciplines are nurtured: research laboratories, medical schools, and hospitals.

The power of these disciplines to dramatically improve the success of twentieth-century medical care is demonstrated, too, in the present content of virtually every medical school curriculum in the United States. These disciplines are assiduously and comprehensively taught during the first two years of medical education, and studiously applied to clinical problems in the last two years. This follows a half-century tradition established since the comprehensive reform of medical education catalyzed by the Flexner Report.

It came as a surprise to Abraham Flexner, a former secondary school administrator and critic of American liberal arts education, when he was asked in 1908 by Henry Prichett, president of the recently established Carnegie Foundation for the Advancement of Teaching, to conduct a study of medical schools in the United States and Canada. Flexner had sought an introduction to Prichett, hoping to find a "congenial

occupation" at the Foundation, and the offer pleased him.
But Flexner believed he was being mistaken for his brother
Simon, a research physician at the Rockefeller Institute.
Dutifully, he told Prichett he was not a doctor, and had never been inside a medical school. "That is precisely what I
want," Prichett replied. "I think these professional
schools should be studied not from the point of view of the
practitioner but from the standpoint of the educator. I know
of your brother, so that I am not laboring under any confu-
sion. This is a layman's job, not a job for a medical man."
(Flexner, 1960)

A foray into the literature on medical education and a
visit to The Johns Hopkins Medical School for discussions
with a number of its famous clinicians were Flexner's prepa-
rations for his tour of the 155 medical schools in the United
States and Canada. His procedure was not that of a modern,
social scientist, survey researcher. He had no question-
naire, only a modest routine of examination. At each school,
he studied the entrance requirements, determined whether
standards announced in the school's catalogue were being followed, and learned the size and training of faculty, the money available to support the institution, the adequacy of laboratories and instruction in basic science, and the relation
between the medical school and its affiliated hospitals.
Several hours were all this estimate usually consumed.

The medical school deans were quite cooperative. They
seemed convinced the Carnegie Foundation was considering
them for an award, despite Flexner's assurances to the con-
trary. Shocking inadequacies passed before Flexner's eyes
as he made his rounds, some of which had a comic aspect. In
Salem, Washington, he asked a dean if his school had a physiology laboratory. "'Surely,'" the dean replied, "'I have it
upstairs. I will bring it to you.'" (Flexner, 1960) He
returned with a sphygmograph, a small device that registers
the motions of the pulse.

Flexner's 1910 report, published in Bulletin Number
Four of the Carnegie Foundation, recommended that the 155
existing medical schools be reduced by 120. Within a decade,
a reduction of nearly this magnitude had taken place. The
fifteen medical schools in Chicago, for example, were conso-
lidated into three.

Not surprisingly, the subjects Flexner emphasized as essential in educating dependable physicians were those then
producing major leaps in the understanding and therapy of
disease. The "medical sciences proper--anatomy, physiology,
pathology, pharmacology" (Flexner, 1910) were to form the

basis of the initial two years of medical school education, with chemistry, physics, and biology proposed as crucial and minimum prerequisites in the course of college study necessary for admission. In an intriguing passage, Flexner acknowledged another aspect of learning important for medical practice--that dealing with social and cultural phenomena. But finding a way to specifically include their study as premedical requirements eluded him. He concluded they would be learned as an aspect of becoming an educated person, and made no special pleas for their specific study (Flexner, 1910).

Only five years before the Flexner Report appeared, a pioneering event had occurred in the integration of the social and cultural aspects of illness into the care of the patient. In 1905, Richard Cabot, a physician at the Massachusetts General Hospital (MGH), introduced the first hospital social service unit in the United States. Its avowed aim was to learn about and treat the social complications of illness through an alliance of physicians and social service workers. The social worker was to bring an understanding of the emotional or social conditions bearing upon the patient's medical condition to the attention of the physician, and jointly design with him an appropriate course of therapy for the patient. Cabot's decision to initiate the unit stemmed from experience as physician to outpatients at the MGH. He became aware that without information about his patient's

> home, about his lodgings, his work, his family, his worries, his nutrition. . . my diagnosis, therefore, remained slipshod and superficial in many cases. . . Treatment in more than half of the cases that I studied involved an understanding of the patient's economic situation and economic means, but still more his mentality, his character, his previous industrial history, all that had brought him to his present condition, in which sickness, fear, worry, and poverty were found inextricably mingled. . . Facing my own failures day after day, seeing my diagnoses useless, not worth the time I had spent in making them because I could not get the necessary treatment carried out, my work came to seem almost intolerable. (Cannon, 1952)

The social service department idea spread throughout American hospitals, and helped to reduce therapeutic mistakes based on poor understanding of the patient's social environment. But by allowing physicians to delegate responsibilities for learning about the social factors, it seems also to have reduced their own need to comprehensively master the knowledge that the social sciences could contribute

to medical care. Further, despite the understanding of the
social dimensions of disease acquired by social workers, a
1943 study revealed that in only a third of American medical
schools were social workers sharing in the teaching, and that
only a handful of this group received official recognition
for their teaching from the school (Cannon, 1952).

Some analysts attributed this problem to the social
worker's limited systematic training in social science research methods and concepts, and to the draining of her time
and energies by large case load and care-taking responsibilities. These circumstances prevented her from adequately representing knowledge of the social sciences to medicine
(Simmons and Wolff, 1954).

The academic-social scientists in this 1940's period
were doing no better than social workers in making their
knowledge useful to medicine. "The related disciplines of
sociology, social psychology, and social anthropology have
been inadequate in concept, research method, and substantive
content for purposes of medical research and practice," noted
the General Director of the Russell Sage Foundation, Donald
Young (Simmons and Wolff, 1954). Part of this problem was
the general inability of social scientists and physicians to
communicate, separated as they were by differences in concepts, methods, technique, and professional jargon; and the
small number of people familiar with both disciplines to help
bridge the interprofessional gaps. Another aspect of the
problem was the difficulty of extracting from the eclectic
theoretical structure of the social sciences the many separate pieces of medically useful knowledge, and singling out
the large number of medical problems that social science research could help solve.

In the mid-1950's, the Flexnerian image of the doctor
as natural scientist continued to prevail in society:

> Every schoolboy who thinks of becoming a physician
> has it quickly impressed on him that he must be
> proficient in chemistry and biology, and perhaps in
> other branches of natural science as well. Patients
> know that the medicines administered to them are
> chemicals and that the technical equipment of hospi-
> tal and private office has been made possible by
> advances in physics, chemistry, and biology. They
> take for granted that the skills of the physician
> are largely the product of knowledge gained from
> the natural sciences. This popular view of modern
> medicine as predominantly biophysical accurately

reflects the overwhelming dependence of current
practice on the natural sciences; it leaves out of
account or minimizes the psychosocial factors in
illness and health. (Simmons and Wolff, 1954)

At this time, however, experts within the medical and
social science communities asserted that a fruitful collabo-
ration between social science and medical science was beginning to take shape. People in both disciplines appeared to
be recognizing problems of shared concern. For example,
growing numbers of social scientists found that the hospital,
the center of medical practice and research, presented them
with an important and fascinating institution to study. And
there was new emphasis in medicine on the social aspects of
some problems, such as the relation of stress and disease:
stress was affected by an individual's perception of a situation; perception in turn was greatly influenced by many
life experiences and cultural and social pressures (Simmons
and Wolff, 1954).

There also were challenges to the often heard claim
that progress in the natural sciences made the social sciences less essential to medicine. Great doctors of past
ages intuitively understood that successful therapy meant
coping with both physical and social dimensions of illness.
But critics declared that relying on intuition was no longer
enough. They called for a systematic effort to unite the
pertinent principles and skills of social and medical science
in caring for the patient.

The effort did not have a significant effect on medical
practice in the 1960's. Wrote one observer:

In spite of improved medical techniques, raised living standards, and more health and welfare legislation, an apparently irreducible mass of sickness re-
mains--minor illnesses, industrial absenteeism, accidents, stress diseases, and the human miseries attend-
ant upon the disruption of house, home and family. . .
Statistics from several industrialized countries
substantiate the existence of a constant mass of
ill-defined sickness. There seems little doubt that
our social pathology is one of the sources of this
ill-health. Its lack of response to current medical
practice and therapy would suggest the desirability
of change in traditional attitudes towards disease
and its causation. Realization that disease does
not always exhibit cellular or biochemical abnorma-
lities is long overdue. (Greenhill, 1961)

The relative security of a biological conception of symptoms, and the relative ease of employing technological solutions to illness, which doctors felt in this period, are gleaned from a clinician's comment on the treatment of diabetes:

A patient comes into the hospital in diabetic coma, and some hot-shot who knows all about chemistry gets him out of coma, regulates his diabetes and sends him back home again; he gets into trouble again, and comes to the medical center every so often. This is a lot of pseudo-science. If you work hard in the medical center, and don't do anything for the felloy when he's home, I don't think this is good. . .[1]

A biological interpretation of disease remains dominant in the 1970's, along with the Flexnerian medical curriculum and the premedical requirements that sustain it. We continue to insist that students preparing for a medical education be required in college to take biology, chemistry, physics, and in some cases, mathematics. There are no specific social science requirements, or humanities requirements for that matter. Such knowledge continues to be viewed in many medical circles as Flexner saw it, sufficiently learned as an aspect of becoming an educated person. One result is that students who are not strong in the sciences, but whose skills and insights into human society, culture, and psychology give them the makings of excellent clinicians, are easily dissuaded from considering a career in medicine.

In most medical schools, the initial two years are dominated by study of the biological sciences. During the clinical years, the medical facts that students and practitioners value most are those derivative of the biological sciences—quantitative and graphically depicted facts generated by the technology of medicine. Information based upon the patient's experience and thoughts about his illness and gathered through history-taking does not receive the same emphasis in medical education or in practice. Thus the facts needed for social science analyses are often inadequately obtained or entirely omitted from a patient's record. Even when diagnostic data bearing upon the socio-cultural aspects of illness are gained, therapeutic actions based on them are often difficult to initiate and sustain. Influencing the social dimensions of an illness often requires the physician to work with people and institutions outside of the hospital. This is time-consuming and requires the physician to step out of his accustomed authoritarian role into one of negotiator. How much more efficient for the physician to initiate biological therapies, and give care in conjunction with people attached to the institution in which he holds power.

I see no comprehensive solution for these problems arising in the near future. But some steps taken now in three directions might help. The social sciences have had their best success in providing physicians with a perspective about cultural and social factors which influence illness. Expanded efforts to do this are clearly warranted. They have been less successful in examining issues of clinical policy, assessing, for example, the outcome of medical interventions in terms of social and cultural variables. Here there is room for more and valuable work. Finally, there is a need to make operational use of the social sciences in direct clinical care; to apply the knowledge of group behavior and dynamics to help physicians gain information from the patient about his illness, and to provide them with new modes of therapy.[2]

To accomplish these objectives, particularly the last, social scientists and physicians must cooperate more fully. The barriers of training and communication between them, described and criticized in the 1940's, still stand, although diminished in size. Each shares responsiblity for their continued existence, and for making new efforts to overcome them.

A biological approach to human illness is a partial approach. It is the task of the social sciences to help demonstrate why, and to participate in initiating the post-Flexnerian era in medicine.

Notes

1. William Soderman cited in J.H. Nodine and J.H. Moyer, eds., Psychosomatic Medicine, Philadelphia: Lea & Feiberger, 1962, 959-960.

2. These distinctions were sharpened in discussions with Dr. John D. Stoeckle of the Massachusetts General Hospital.

References

Cannon, Ida M. On the Social Frontier of Medicine. Cambridge, Mass.: Harvard University Press, 1952.

Flexner, Abraham. Abraham Flexner: An Autobiography. New York: Simon and Schuster, 1960.

Flexner, Abraham. Medical Education in the United States and Canada. New York: Carnegie Foundation for the Advancement of Teaching, Bulletin No. 4, 1910.

Greenhill, Stanley. "Industrialization: Its Challenge to Medicine." Lancet, 1 (1961): 1182.

Holmes, Oliver Wendell. "Currents and Counter-Currents in Medical Science." In Medical Essays. Boston: Houghton, Mifflin and Co., 1883.

Nodine, J.H. and J.H. Moyer, eds. Psychosomatic Medicine. Philadelphia: Lea & Feiberger, 1962.

Simmons, Leo W. and Harold G. Wolff. Social Science in Medicine. New York: Russell Sage Foundation, 1954.